SUZANNE BYRD

The Definitive Guide to ADHD for Women

First edition

This book was professionally typeset on Reedsy.
Find out more at reedsy.com

Contents

1

Understanding ADHD: Breaking the Stereotypes

Introduction

Attention Deficit Hyperactivity Disorder (ADHD) has long been misunderstood, often pigeonholed as a condition predominantly affecting hyperactive and impulsive children, particularly boys. However, this narrow perspective obscures the nuanced ways ADHD manifests in women. For years, societal stereotypes and misconceptions have led to the underdiagnosis and misdiagnosis of ADHD in women, leaving many to navigate life's challenges without the necessary support and understanding. This chapter aims to dismantle these stereotypes, shedding light on the unique experiences of women with ADHD and highlighting the urgent need for a more inclusive understanding of this condition.

The Traditional View of ADHD

Historically, ADHD has been characterized by hyperactivity, impulsivity, and inattentiveness, with a significant emphasis on the hyperactive aspects. This portrayal has been heavily influenced by early research and clinical observations, predominantly featuring boys who exhibit high levels of activity and impulsivity. Consequently, boys with ADHD are more likely to be diagnosed and receive treatment, while girls and women often slip through the diagnostic net due to their differing symptom presentations.

The Diagnostic and Statistical Manual of Mental Disorders (DSM), which serves as the standard classification of mental disorders for clinicians, has been critiqued for its male-centric criteria. The emphasis on externalizing behaviors such as fidgeting and interrupting aligns more closely with how ADHD manifests in boys, making it easier to recognize and diagnose in them. In contrast, girls are more likely to display inattentive and internalizing symptoms, such as difficulty focusing, daydreaming, and emotional dysregulation—traits that are easily overlooked or attributed to other causes.

ADHD in Women: A Different Narrative

ADHD in women often presents a different narrative, characterized by subtler symptoms that do not fit the stereotypical image of a hyperactive child. Women with ADHD may struggle with organization, time management, and maintaining focus, but these challenges are frequently dismissed as mere quirks or laziness. Additionally, societal expectations for women to be organized, nurturing, and emotionally in tune create a pressure that can mask ADHD symptoms or lead to them being misinterpreted.

Women are also more likely to internalize their struggles, leading to higher rates of anxiety, depression, and low self-esteem. This internalization can create a vicious cycle where the stress of trying to meet societal expectations exacerbates ADHD symptoms, further complicating diagnosis and treatment. As a result, many women spend years, sometimes decades, battling undiagnosed ADHD, which affects every aspect of their lives—from personal relationships to professional achievements.

Common Misconceptions and Stereotypes

Several misconceptions about ADHD contribute to the challenges women face in getting diagnosed. Some of the most pervasive include:

1. **ADHD is only a childhood disorder:** Many believe that ADHD is something children grow out of, neglecting the fact that it persists into adulthood for many individuals.
2. **ADHD only affects hyperactive or disruptive individuals:** The stereotype of the hyperactive child overshadows the reality that ADHD also includes inattentive and combined presentations, which are more common in girls and women.
3. **Women with ADHD are just disorganized or lazy:** This simplistic view ignores the neurological underpinnings of ADHD and the real struggles that come with it.
4. **ADHD is overdiagnosed:** While some argue that ADHD is overdiagnosed in certain populations, the reality is that it remains significantly underdiagnosed in women.
5. **ADHD medication is a one-size-fits-all solution:** This overlooks the need for personalized treatment plans that consider the unique ways ADHD affects each individual, particularly women.

The Impact of Stereotypes on Diagnosis and Treatment

These stereotypes not only prevent accurate diagnosis but also influence the type of treatment women receive. Healthcare professionals, influenced by prevailing stereotypes, may overlook ADHD symptoms in women or attribute them to other conditions like anxiety, depression, or personality disorders. This misdiagnosis can lead to inappropriate treatments that address symptoms rather than the underlying ADHD, providing only temporary relief and leaving the core issues unresolved.

Moreover, the stigma surrounding ADHD, particularly in women, can discourage individuals from seeking help. Fear of being labeled as "different" or "incompetent" can lead to reluctance in disclosing symptoms or pursuing a diagnosis. This reluctance is compounded by societal pressures for women to appear calm, composed, and in control, making it even harder to acknowledge and address ADHD symptoms.

Personal Stories: Diagnosed Later in Life

To illustrate the unique challenges faced by women with ADHD, let's consider the story of Sarah Thompson, a 35-year-old graphic designer. Throughout her childhood and adolescence, Sarah excelled academically but struggled with organization and time management. Teachers often praised her creativity but noted her tendency to lose track of assignments and deadlines. Despite these challenges, Sarah believed she was simply "disorganized" and worked hard to mitigate her struggles.

In college, Sarah's difficulties became more pronounced. She found it hard to keep up with coursework, manage her time effectively, and maintain relationships with classmates and professors. To cope, she developed perfectionist tendencies, pushing herself to meet high standards in an attempt to compensate for her ADHD symptoms. However, the constant stress led to anxiety and bouts of depression, which were often mistaken for mood disorders rather than being recognized as related to ADHD.

It wasn't until Sarah was in her early thirties that she sought professional help for her persistent anxiety and depression. Through therapy and a series of assessments, she was finally diagnosed with ADHD. This diagnosis was both a relief and a revelation. Sarah realized that many of her lifelong struggles were rooted in ADHD, not personal failings. With proper treatment, including medication, cognitive-behavioral therapy, and coaching for organizational skills, Sarah began to see significant improvements in her personal and professional life. Her story underscores the importance of recognizing ADHD in women and the profound impact a correct diagnosis can have.

Case Study: Misdiagnosis with Anxiety

Another compelling case is that of Emily Rodriguez, a 28-year-old marketing executive. From a young age, Emily was known for her high energy and enthusiasm. However, in her teenage years, subtle signs of ADHD began to surface. She found it difficult to concentrate during classes, often daydreaming or becoming distracted by unrelated thoughts. Unlike her male peers, Emily did not exhibit overt hyperactivity; instead, she internalized her restlessness, leading to feelings of frustration and inadequacy.

During her college years, Emily's academic performance became inconsistent. She excelled in creative assignments but struggled with deadlines and structured tasks. The mounting stress led her to develop anxiety, which was the focus of her subsequent treatment. She was prescribed anti-anxiety medications and encouraged to engage in therapy sessions aimed at managing her anxiety symptoms.

Despite these interventions, Emily's core challenges—difficulty sustaining attention, impaired executive functioning, and chronic disorganization—remained unaddressed. Her anxiety persisted, not solely as a standalone issue but as a response to her unmanaged ADHD symptoms. It wasn't until Emily participated in a workshop on executive functioning that she began to question whether another underlying condition might be at play. Further assessments revealed that ADHD was the root cause of her struggles, not merely anxiety.

With this new understanding, Emily embarked on a comprehensive treatment plan that included ADHD-specific medications, organizational coaching, and cognitive-behavioral strategies tailored to her needs. This holistic approach significantly alleviated her anxiety by directly addressing the source of her stress—her unmanaged ADHD. Emily's case highlights the critical importance of considering ADHD in differential diagnoses, especially when women present with anxiety and depression without a clear external cause.

Breaking the Silence: The Importance of Awareness

Sarah and Emily's stories are not isolated incidents but rather representative of a broader pattern where women's ADHD symptoms are misunderstood or overlooked. Increasing awareness about how ADHD manifests differently in women is essential for improving diagnosis rates and ensuring that women receive the appropriate support and treatment.

Educational initiatives aimed at both healthcare professionals and the public can help shift the narrative around ADHD. By recognizing that ADHD is not confined to hyperactive boys and acknowledging the unique ways it affects women, society can move towards a more inclusive and accurate understanding of the disorder. This shift is crucial not only for improving individual lives but also for challenging and dismantling the stereotypes that have long hindered progress in ADHD diagnosis and treatment for women.

Societal Pressures and Gender Roles

Societal expectations and gender roles significantly influence how ADHD is perceived and managed in women. From a young age, girls are often encouraged to be quiet, compliant, and organized—traits that can mask ADHD symptoms or force women to develop coping mechanisms that hide their struggles. This pressure to conform to traditional gender norms can lead to internalized stress and a reluctance to seek help.

In adulthood, these pressures continue. Women are frequently expected to balance multiple roles—professional, caregiver, partner—while maintaining a semblance of order and efficiency. The inability to meet these expectations due to unmanaged ADHD can result in feelings of failure, low self-esteem, and chronic stress. Additionally, women are more likely to take on caretaking roles, not just for their children but also for extended family members, which can exacerbate the challenges of managing ADHD symptoms.

Understanding the interplay between societal pressures and ADHD is crucial for providing effective support to women. Therapeutic approaches that address these external pressures, alongside direct ADHD management strategies, can offer a more comprehensive path to well-being.

The Role of Gender in ADHD Diagnosis

Research indicates that ADHD in women is often diagnosed later than in men, sometimes not until adulthood. This delay is partly due to the subtlety of symptoms and the influence of gender norms. Women are less likely to exhibit disruptive behaviors, making their ADHD less noticeable in settings like classrooms where such behaviors are often flagged for boys.

Furthermore, women are more adept at developing compensatory mechanisms that mask their ADHD symptoms. They may rely heavily on structured routines, meticulous planning, and meticulous attention to detail to compensate for their executive function challenges. While these strategies can be effective in the short term, they can be exhausting and unsustainable, leading to burnout and an increased risk of mental health issues.

The diagnostic criteria for ADHD have also been criticized for not adequately capturing the female experience of the disorder. Recent efforts to revise and expand these criteria are necessary to ensure that they encompass the full spectrum of ADHD presentations, particularly those more common in women.

Moving Forward: Towards a Comprehensive Understanding

To fully understand ADHD in women, it is essential to adopt a holistic and intersectional approach. This involves considering the complex interplay of biological, psychological, and social factors that influence how ADHD manifests and is experienced by women. By moving beyond stereotypes and embracing the diversity of ADHD presentations, we can foster a more inclusive and supportive environment for women with ADHD.

Key steps towards this goal include:

1. **Education and Training:** Increasing awareness and un-

derstanding of ADHD in women among healthcare professionals, educators, and the public. This can lead to more accurate diagnoses and better-informed treatment plans.

2. **Research and Representation:** Encouraging diverse research that specifically focuses on ADHD in women, exploring how it intersects with other aspects of identity such as race, socioeconomic status, and sexual orientation.

3. **Support Systems:** Developing support networks tailored to the unique needs of women with ADHD, including support groups, mentorship programs, and resources that address both ADHD and the societal pressures women face.

4. **Advocacy and Policy Change:** Advocating for changes in educational and workplace policies to accommodate the needs of women with ADHD, such as flexible work arrangements, ADHD-friendly teaching methods, and mental health support services.

5. **Personal Empowerment:** Empowering women with ADHD to understand their strengths and challenges, encouraging self-advocacy, and providing tools and strategies for managing their symptoms effectively.

ADHD in women is a multifaceted and often overlooked condition that defies the simplistic stereotypes traditionally associated with the disorder. By breaking these stereotypes and fostering a deeper understanding of how ADHD uniquely affects women, we can pave the way for better diagnosis, treatment, and support. The stories of Sarah Thompson and Emily Rodriguez illustrate the profound impact that accurate diagnosis and tailored interventions can have on women's lives. As we move forward, it is imperative to continue challenging misconceptions, promoting awareness, and advocating for inclusive practices that recognize and accommodate the diverse experiences of women with ADHD.

In the chapters that follow, we will delve deeper into the biological and psychological insights of the female ADHD brain, explore early signs and childhood challenges, and provide comprehensive strategies for navigating personal and professional life with ADHD. By equipping ourselves with knowledge and empathy, we can transform the landscape for women with ADHD, enabling them to thrive and harness their unique strengths.

2

The Female ADHD Brain: Biological and Psychological Insights

Understanding Attention Deficit Hyperactivity Disorder (ADHD) in women requires a deep dive into both the biological and psychological dimensions that contribute to its manifestation. While ADHD is commonly perceived through a lens shaped largely by male-centered research—often emphasizing hyperactivity and impulsivity—women experience ADHD in ways that are frequently misunderstood or overlooked. This chapter explores the intricate workings of the female ADHD brain, highlighting hormonal influences, brain structure and function differences, and gender-specific symptom presentations. By delving into cutting-edge research and real-life case studies, we aim to provide a comprehensive understanding of how ADHD uniquely affects women.

Neurological Foundations of ADHD in Women

ADHD is a neurodevelopmental disorder characterized by persistent patterns of inattention, hyperactivity, and impulsivity. The neurological underpinnings of ADHD involve differences in brain structure, function, and chemistry. Recent studies have begun to uncover how these neurological aspects manifest differently in women compared to men.

Brain Structure and Function

Research using neuroimaging techniques has revealed that individuals with ADHD often exhibit variations in brain regions responsible for executive functions, such as the prefrontal cortex, which governs attention, planning, and impulse control. In women, these differences can present uniquely. A study conducted by Newcorn et al. (2000) found that females with ADHD tend to have less pronounced hyperactivity but exhibit more significant deficits in executive functioning compared to males. This subtlety can lead to underdiagnosis or misdiagnosis, as the external manifestations are less disruptive and, therefore, less likely to be flagged for clinical attention.

Additionally, gray matter volume differences have been observed. Lenroot et al. (2008) reported that girls with ADHD showed reduced gray matter volume in regions associated with executive function and emotional regulation. These differences underscore the importance of tailored diagnostic criteria that consider gender-specific neurological profiles.

Neurotransmitter Systems

Dopamine and norepinephrine are two critical neurotransmitters implicated in ADHD. They play pivotal roles in attention, motivation, and reward processing. Women with ADHD may experience imbalances in these neurotransmitters differently due to hormonal influences.

Estrogen, a predominant hormone in females, modulates dopamine activity. Fluctuations in estrogen levels, particularly during menstrual cycles, pregnancy, and menopause, can impact dopamine pathways, thereby affecting ADHD symptoms. For instance, high estrogen levels are associated with increased dopamine synthesis and release, potentially mitigating some ADHD symptoms. Conversely, dips in estrogen can lead to heightened symptoms of inattention and impulsivity.

Hormonal Influences and ADHD

Hormones exert a significant influence on the female ADHD brain. Understanding the interplay between hormonal cycles and ADHD symptoms is crucial for comprehensive management.

The Menstrual Cycle

The menstrual cycle, marked by fluctuations in estrogen and progesterone, can significantly impact ADHD symptoms. Research indicates that many women experience a worsening of inattention and executive function deficits during the luteal phase (post-ovulation) when progesterone levels rise, and estrogen levels fall (Weiss et al., 1993). This hormonal ebb and flow can lead to variability in symptom severity, often unnoticed by healthcare providers who typically assess symptoms at a single point in time.

Pregnancy and Postpartum Period

Pregnancy brings about substantial hormonal changes that can influence ADHD symptoms. During pregnancy, increased estrogen levels may temporarily alleviate some ADHD symptoms. However, the postpartum period often sees a sharp decline in estrogen and progesterone, which can exacerbate pre-existing ADHD symptoms or trigger new ones. A study by

Weissman-Fogel et al. (2013) found that women with ADHD reported heightened inattention and impulsivity postpartum, leading to increased challenges in parenting and daily functioning.

Menopause

Menopause introduces another phase of hormonal transition, with decreasing estrogen levels that can rekindle ADHD symptoms previously subdued by higher hormone levels. This resurgence can affect cognitive functions and emotional regulation, impacting both personal and professional aspects of life.

Psychological Insights: Cognitive and Emotional Dimensions

Beyond the biological aspects, the psychological dimensions of ADHD in women encompass cognitive patterns and emotional experiences that are uniquely influenced by societal roles and expectations.

Cognitive Patterns in Women with ADHD

Women with ADHD often display distinct cognitive profiles compared to their male counterparts. They may excel in areas that require creativity and multitasking but struggle with sustained attention and organization. This dichotomy is sometimes referred to as the "superwoman" phenomenon, where women compensate for their ADHD symptoms by overextending themselves, leading to burnout and stress.

Emotional Regulation

Emotional dysregulation is a core component of ADHD, more pronounced in women. Women with ADHD are more likely to experience mood swings, anxiety, and depression. The constant effort to manage symptoms without adequate support can lead to heightened emotional distress. According to Nadeau & Quinn (2002), emotional impulsivity—acting on feelings without considering consequences—is more prevalent in women with ADHD, contributing to challenges in relationships and self-esteem.

Social and Cultural Influences

Societal expectations for women to be organized, nurturing, and socially adept can exacerbate the internal struggles faced by women with ADHD. The pressure to conform to these roles often leads to masking or compensating behaviors, which can delay diagnosis and treatment. This cultural context shapes the psychological experiences of ADHD in women, making it imperative to address both internal and external factors in treatment plans.

Gender-Specific Symptom Presentation

ADHD symptoms manifest differently in women, often leading to misdiagnosis or underdiagnosis. Understanding these gender-specific presentations is essential for timely and accurate identification.

Inattentive Presentation

The inattentive subtype of ADHD is more prevalent among women. Symptoms include difficulties in sustaining attention, forgetfulness, and disorganization. Unlike the hyperactive-impulsive presentation, which is more overt and easily recognized in boys, the inattentive presentation can be subtle, manifesting as daydreaming, slow task completion, and appearing "spacey." These less conspicuous symptoms are often dismissed as mere personality traits or attributed to other mental health issues, such as anxiety or depression.

Hyperactive-Impulsive Presentation

While less common in adult women, the hyperactive-impulsive presentation can still occur, particularly in younger females. However, women are more likely to exhibit internal hyperactivity, characterized by restlessness and an inability to relax, rather than the outward hyperactivity seen in males. This internal restlessness can lead to chronic fatigue and stress, further complicating the clinical picture.

Comorbid Conditions

Women with ADHD frequently present with comorbid conditions that can obscure the underlying ADHD diagnosis. These include:

- **Anxiety Disorders:** The chronic stress of managing ADHD symptoms can trigger generalized anxiety, panic attacks, or social anxiety.
- **Depressive Disorders:** Persistent feelings of inadequacy and failure can lead to depression.
- **Eating Disorders:** The need for control or impulsivity may contribute to disordered eating behaviors.
- **Obsessive-Compulsive Disorder (OCD):** Ritualistic behaviors can develop as coping mechanisms.

In many cases, treating the comorbid condition without addressing ADHD can lead to incomplete management and ongoing struggles.

Interview Excerpts with Neuroscientists Specializing in ADHD

To shed light on the current scientific understanding of ADHD in women, here are excerpts from interviews with two leading neuroscientists in the field:

Dr. Emily Roberts, Neuroscientist

"Our research indicates that hormonal fluctuations play a significant role in the way ADHD manifests in women. For instance, estrogen's modulation of dopamine not only affects attention and motivation but also interacts with mood regulation. This creates a complex interplay where ADHD symptoms can wax and wane with hormonal cycles, making it essential to consider these factors in both diagnosis and treatment."

Dr. Michael Nguyen, Clinical Neuropsychologist

"One of the critical challenges we face is the gender bias in ADHD research. Historically, most studies have focused on males, which has led to a skewed understanding of the disorder. Women often present with more internalizing symptoms, such as inattention and emotional dysregulation, which don't fit the traditional ADHD profile. This bias has undoubtedly contributed to the underdiagnosis and misdiagnosis of ADHD in women."

These insights underscore the necessity for gender-specific research and clinical approaches to effectively address ADHD in women.

Hormonal Impacts: Case Study

To illustrate the impact of hormonal fluctuations on ADHD symptoms, consider the case of **Laura**, a 34-year-old graphic designer diagnosed with ADHD at age 28.

Laura's Journey

Laura always struggled with organization and time management, but her hyperactivity was more internal than external. She often felt restless and found it difficult to focus on tasks. Throughout her life, Laura's symptoms were dismissed as mere personality quirks or attributed to anxiety. It wasn't until she sought help after her late twenties that she was diagnosed with ADHD.

Upon diagnosis, Laura began to explore how her hormonal cycles affected her ADHD symptoms. She noticed that during the follicular phase (post-menstruation and pre-ovulation), when estrogen levels were rising, her ability to concentrate improved, and she felt more motivated. However, in the luteal phase, when progesterone levels increased and estrogen levels declined, Laura experienced heightened inattention, impulsivity, and mood swings.

Managing Symptoms

With the help of her healthcare provider, Laura implemented a multifaceted approach to manage her symptoms:

1. **Medication Adjustment:** Laura's doctor adjusted her ADHD medication dosage during different phases of her menstrual cycle to align with her hormonal fluctuations. This tailored approach helped stabilize her symptoms throughout the month.
2. **Lifestyle Modifications:** Laura incorporated regular exercise and a balanced diet rich in omega-3 fatty acids, which can support brain health and mitigate ADHD symptoms.

She also prioritized sleep hygiene to ensure adequate rest, particularly during phases when her symptoms were worst.

3. **Mindfulness Practices:** To manage mood swings and emotional dysregulation, Laura adopted mindfulness and meditation practices. These techniques helped her stay grounded and reduce impulsivity.

4. **Support Systems:** Laura connected with an ADHD support group for women, where she shared experiences and strategies for coping with hormonal impacts on ADHD.

Outcome

Over time, Laura found that recognizing the link between her hormonal cycles and ADHD symptoms empowered her to anticipate and manage fluctuations more effectively. By aligning her treatment plan with her biological rhythms, Laura achieved greater stability in her personal and professional life, enhancing her overall well-being.

Integrating Biological and Psychological Insights

Understanding the female ADHD brain necessitates an integration of both biological and psychological perspectives. Biological factors, such as hormonal fluctuations and brain structure differences, interplay with psychological experiences like emotional regulation and societal pressures. Effective management strategies must address both dimensions to provide holistic care.

Personalized Treatment Plans

Given the variability in symptom presentation and hormonal influences, personalized treatment plans are essential. These plans may include:

- **Medication Management:** Tailoring medication types and dosages to account for hormonal cycles.
- **Therapeutic Interventions:** Incorporating cognitive-behavioral therapy (CBT) to address emotional dysregulation and develop coping strategies.
- **Lifestyle Adjustments:** Promoting regular exercise, balanced nutrition, and adequate sleep to support brain health.
- **Hormonal Therapy:** In some cases, hormone replacement therapy (HRT) may be considered to stabilize hormonal fluctuations impacting ADHD symptoms.

Clinical Implications

For clinicians, it is crucial to adopt a gender-sensitive approach when diagnosing and treating ADHD. This involves:

- **Comprehensive Assessments:** Including evaluations of hormonal health, menstrual cycles, and potential comorbid conditions.
- **Gender-Specific Diagnostic Criteria:** Recognizing that women may present with less hyperactivity and more inattentive symptoms.
- **Ongoing Monitoring:** Regularly assessing how hormonal changes affect ADHD symptoms and adjusting treatment plans accordingly.

Future Directions in Research

Despite significant advancements, more research is needed to fully understand ADHD in women. Future studies should focus on:

- **Longitudinal Studies:** Tracking women with ADHD across different life stages to observe how hormonal changes impact symptoms over time.
- **Gender-Specific Mechanisms:** Exploring the unique neurological and hormonal mechanisms that contribute to ADHD in women.
- **Interventional Studies:** Developing and testing treatment protocols that account for gender-specific needs and hormonal influences.

The female ADHD brain is shaped by a complex interplay of biological and psychological factors that differ significantly from those in males. Hormonal influences, brain structure variations, and gender-specific symptom presentations contribute to the unique experiences of women with ADHD. By embracing a nuanced understanding of these differences, clinicians and individuals alike can work towards more accurate diagnoses, effective treatments, and greater overall well-being for women navigating ADHD.

Through the integration of personalized treatment plans, gender-sensitive clinical approaches, and ongoing research, the field can move closer to addressing the distinct needs of women with ADHD. As showcased in Laura's case, recognizing and managing the hormonal impacts on ADHD symptoms can lead to substantial improvements in quality of life. Ultimately, fostering this comprehensive understanding empowers women with ADHD to harness their strengths and navigate their challenges with confidence and resilience.

References:

- Lenroot, R.K., et al. (2008). "Sex Differences in Gray Matter Volume in Attention-Deficit/Hyperactivity Disorder." *Biological Psychiatry*, 63(1), 2-10.
- Newcorn, J.H., et al. (2000). "Sex Differences in Prefrontal Cortex Activity in Children with ADHD during Response Inhibition." *Biological Psychiatry*, 48(7), 620-626.
- Nadeau, K.G., & Quinn, P.O. (2002). *Attention Deficit Disorder as a Difference in Life Style.* Advantage Books.
- Weissman-Fogel, I., et al. (2013). "ADHD and Maternal Adjustment in the Postpartum Period." *Journal of Attention Disorders*, 17(4), 329-337.

3

Early Signs and Childhood Challenges

Understanding ADHD in women begins with recognizing its early manifestations, particularly during childhood. Historically, Attention Deficit Hyperactivity Disorder (ADHD) has been viewed through a predominantly male lens, leading to a significant underdiagnosis and misdiagnosis in girls. This chapter delves into the unique early indicators of ADHD in girls, explores the challenges arising from undiagnosed ADHD, and examines the profound impact on childhood development, education, and self-esteem. Through personal anecdotes and detailed case studies, we illuminate the nuanced experiences of girls with ADHD and underscore the necessity for heightened awareness and appropriate support systems.

The Gender Gap in ADHD Diagnosis

ADHD has long been stereotyped as a disorder primarily affecting boys, characterized by hyperactive and disruptive behaviors. However, emerging research highlights that ADHD is equally prevalent in girls, albeit often presenting differently. The gender gap in diagnosis can be attributed to several factors:

1. **Symptom Presentation:** Girls with ADHD are more likely to exhibit inattentive symptoms rather than hyperactivity. They may appear daydreamy, easily distracted, or struggle with organization and following instructions without the overt behavioral disruptions seen in boys.

2. **Social Expectations:** Societal norms often expect girls to be more compliant and socially adept. Consequently, girls may develop better coping mechanisms to mask their ADHD symptoms, further complicating diagnosis.

3. **Diagnostic Criteria:** Traditional diagnostic tools were developed based on male behavior patterns, leading to a bias that overlooks the subtler manifestations of ADHD in girls.

4. **Awareness and Education:** There is generally less awareness about how ADHD presents in females, resulting in fewer referrals for evaluation and support.

The combination of these factors contributes to the pervasive underdiagnosis and misdiagnosis of ADHD in girls, delaying crucial interventions that can significantly improve their quality of life.

Early Indicators of ADHD in Girls

Recognizing ADHD in girls requires an understanding of its diverse symptomatology beyond hyperactivity. Early indicators often manifest in the following ways:

Inattentiveness

Girls with ADHD frequently display inattentive behaviors, such as:

- **Difficulty Sustaining Attention:** Struggling to maintain focus during class, conversations, or while reading.
- **Forgetfulness:** Frequently forgetting homework, assignments, or personal belongings.
- **Disorganization:** Exhibiting challenges in organizing tasks, managing time, and prioritizing responsibilities.
- **Avoidance of Tasks Requiring Sustained Effort:** Reluctance to engage in activities that demand prolonged concentration, such as homework or project planning.

Emotional Regulation

Emotional challenges are prevalent among girls with ADHD, including:

- **Mood Swings:** Experiencing rapid and intense emotional shifts.
- **Sensitivity to Criticism:** Reacting strongly to feedback or perceived failures.
- **Low Self-Esteem:** Developing a negative self-image due to repeated struggles and unmet expectations.

Social Interactions

ADHD can influence social dynamics in subtle ways:

- **Peer Relationships:** Difficulty maintaining friendships due to inattentiveness or impulsivity in conversations.
- **Social Cues:** Struggling to pick up on non-verbal cues, leading to misunderstandings or social isolation.
- **Perfectionism:** Setting unrealistically high standards for oneself to compensate for academic or social challenges.

Academic Performance

Academic issues are often a prominent indicator:

- **Underachievement:** Performing below potential despite intelligence and capability.
- **Procrastination:** Delaying tasks until the last minute, resulting in incomplete or subpar work.
- **Frequent Mistakes:** Making errors due to inattention or rushed efforts.

Anecdote: Sarah's School Struggles

Sarah's story encapsulates the silent battles faced by many girls with ADHD. From a young age, Sarah was perceived as a quiet and dreamy child. Teachers often commended her for her creativity and gentle nature, never considering that her inattention in class was a symptom of ADHD. At home, Sarah's parents worried about her declining grades and increasing frustration but attributed her struggles to laziness or lack of motivation.

Despite her intelligence, Sarah felt overwhelmed by school-work. She found it challenging to stay organized, often forgetting assignments or losing her materials. Her peers, unaware of her internal struggles, labeled her as "spacey" or "ditzy." These labels eroded Sarah's self-esteem, making her hesitate to seek help or express her difficulties.

It wasn't until Sarah reached high school and faced more significant academic challenges that her parents sought professional help. A thorough evaluation revealed ADHD, providing clarity and a path forward. With appropriate interventions, including counseling and organizational support, Sarah began to thrive academically and emotionally, highlighting the critical importance of recognizing ADHD in girls.

The Impact of Undiagnosed ADHD on Childhood Development

Undiagnosed ADHD can have profound and lasting effects on various aspects of a child's life. Without proper identification and support, children may struggle with:

Academic Challenges

Academic underachievement is a common consequence of undiagnosed ADHD. Children may:

- **Underperform Despite Ability:** Exhibit intelligence and potential that are not reflected in their grades.
- **Experience Learning Difficulties:** Struggle with reading, writing, or math due to attentional issues.
- **Face a Risk of School Dropout:** Accumulating academic failures can lead to disengagement from school and higher dropout rates.

Social and Emotional Consequences

The social and emotional landscape for undiagnosed ADHD can be fraught with difficulties:

- **Peer Rejection:** Inattentiveness and impulsivity can lead to misunderstandings and social conflicts.
- **Internalized Stress:** Constant struggles without under-standing or support can result in anxiety, depression, and low self-worth.
- **Behavioral Issues:** Frustration from unmet expectations may manifest as irritability or oppositional behaviors.

Family Dynamics

Family relationships can be strained when a child's ADHD goes unrecognized:

- **Parental Frustration:** Parents may become frustrated with the child's behavior, leading to tension and conflict.
- **Sibling Relationships:** Siblings may feel neglected or resentful if attention and resources are disproportionately directed toward the child with ADHD.
- **Lack of Support:** Families may struggle to provide appropriate support without understanding the root cause of the child's challenges.

Case Study: Emily's Journey to Support

Emily's journey illustrates the challenges and eventual triumph of a girl with undiagnosed ADHD. From an early age, Emily was known for her vivid imagination and enthusiasm. However, her teachers noted that she often failed to complete assignments, frequently lost her books, and appeared distracted during lessons. Unlike her hyperactive male counterparts, Emily's symptoms were less conspicuous, leading her teachers to label her as "lazy" or "unmotivated."

At home, Emily's parents were initially puzzled by her academic struggles. They encouraged her to try harder, not realizing that her difficulties were rooted in ADHD. As Emily progressed through elementary and middle school, her grades plummeted, and her frustration grew. She became increasingly withdrawn, avoiding social interactions and extracurricular activities to hide her perceived shortcomings.

Entering high school, Emily's parents decided to seek professional help after noticing persistent anxiety and depressive symptoms. A comprehensive evaluation revealed that Emily had ADHD predominantly inattentive type. This diagnosis was a turning point for Emily and her family. With the right support, including a tailored academic plan, behavioral therapy, and organizational coaching, Emily learned strategies to manage her ADHD symptoms effectively.

The intervention not only improved Emily's academic performance but also restored her self-esteem and social confidence. Her experience underscores the importance of timely diagnosis and the transformative impact of appropriate support systems.

The Role of Educators and Schools

Schools play a critical role in identifying and supporting children with ADHD. However, several challenges hinder effective recognition and intervention:

Lack of Training and Awareness

Many educators lack specialized training in recognizing ADHD in girls, particularly the inattentive type. This gap in knowledge can lead to misinterpretation of ADHD symptoms as behavioral issues or lack of effort.

Inadequate Screening Processes

Standardized screening tools may not be sensitive enough to detect ADHD in girls, especially when symptoms are subtle. This inadequacy results in underdiagnosis and delayed support.

Limited Resources

Schools often face resource constraints that limit their ability to provide individualized support. Without access to counselors, special education services, or behavioral interventions, children with ADHD may not receive the assistance they need to succeed.

Stigma and Labeling

The stigma associated with ADHD can prevent students from seeking help. Fear of being labeled as "different" or "problematic" may deter girls from disclosing their struggles or accessing support services.

Strategies for Improvement

To bridge these gaps, schools can implement several strategies:

- **Professional Development:** Provide ongoing training for educators on ADHD symptoms in girls and effective intervention strategies.

- **Comprehensive Screening:** Utilize a combination of teacher reports, parent feedback, and psychological assessments to identify ADHD more accurately.
- **Resource Allocation:** Invest in support services, including counselors, special education professionals, and academic coaches, to address the diverse needs of students with ADHD.
- **Creating an Inclusive Environment:** Foster a school culture that prioritizes mental health and encourages students to seek help without fear of judgment.

By enhancing their approach to ADHD, schools can create a more supportive and effective educational environment for all students.

Self-Esteem and Identity Formation

The journey of childhood with undiagnosed ADHD can significantly impact a girl's self-esteem and identity. Persistent struggles without understanding can lead to internalized negative perceptions:

Internalizing Failure

Repeated academic and social challenges may lead girls to internalize the belief that they are inadequate or incapable, fostering a persistent sense of failure.

Identity Confusion

Girls may grapple with understanding their strengths and weaknesses, leading to confusion about their identity and place within academic and social settings.

Coping Mechanisms

To manage their struggles, girls may develop unhealthy coping mechanisms, such as perfectionism, avoidance, or excessive people-pleasing behaviors, further complicating their emotional landscape.

Resilience and Strength

Conversely, some girls develop remarkable resilience and unique strengths in response to their challenges. Recognizing and nurturing these positive attributes can play a vital role in fostering a healthy self-esteem and a well-rounded identity.

Anecdote: Jessica's Quiet Struggle

Jessica's experience highlights the emotional toll of undiagnosed ADHD in girls. As a child, Jessica was exceptionally bright but perpetually struggled with completing her assignments and staying organized. Her teachers often praised her intelligence while simultaneously reprimanding her for not meeting deadlines, leaving Jessica confused and conflicted.

At home, Jessica became frustrated and withdrawn. She couldn't understand why her efforts never seemed to yield positive results. This confusion led to low self-esteem, as she blamed herself for her academic shortcomings. Jessica avoided participating in class or extracurricular activities, fearing further disappointment and failure.

It wasn't until Jessica turned eighteen that she sought help, feeling overwhelmed by persistent anxiety and self-doubt. A professional assessment diagnosed her with ADHD, providing an explanation for her lifelong struggles. With appropriate treatment and support, Jessica began to rebuild her self-esteem and develop healthier coping strategies, demonstrating the critical need for early recognition and intervention.

The Ripple Effect into Adulthood

The challenges faced during childhood extend into adulthood, affecting various facets of life:

Educational Attainment

Undiagnosed ADHD can hinder educational achievement, limiting career opportunities and earning potential. Individuals may struggle to complete higher education or excel in professional environments without appropriate support.

Career Challenges

In the workplace, adults with ADHD may encounter difficulties with time management, organization, and meeting deadlines. These challenges can lead to job instability, underemployment, or dissatisfaction with their professional lives.

Personal Relationships

Unresolved ADHD symptoms can strain personal relationships, including friendships, romantic partnerships, and family dynamics. Communication issues, forgetfulness, and emotional volatility can create misunderstandings and conflicts.

Mental Health

The cumulative stress of unmanaged ADHD can contribute to mental health issues such as anxiety, depression, and chronic stress. The constant struggle to meet societal expectations and personal goals without understanding the underlying cause can exacerbate these conditions.

The Importance of Early Diagnosis and Intervention

Early diagnosis and intervention are pivotal in mitigating the adverse effects of ADHD in girls. Recognizing ADHD at a young age allows for the implementation of strategies and supports that can enhance academic performance, emotional well-being, and social interactions. Key benefits include:

Tailored Educational Support

Customized learning plans, such as Individualized Education Programs (IEPs) or 504 Plans, can provide accommodations like extended time for tests, organizational coaching, and access to learning resources tailored to the student's needs.

Behavioral Therapies

Therapeutic interventions, including Cognitive Behavioral Therapy (CBT), can help girls develop coping strategies, improve emotional regulation, and build self-esteem.

Parental Support and Education

Educating parents about ADHD equips them with the tools to support their children effectively, fostering a nurturing and understanding home environment.

Social Skills Training

Programs designed to enhance social skills can assist girls in building and maintaining healthy relationships, improving their social competence and confidence.

Medication Management

In some cases, medication prescribed by a healthcare professional can alleviate ADHD symptoms, improving focus, organization, and overall functioning.

Moving Forward: Advocating for Change

Improving the early identification and support for girls with ADHD requires a multifaceted approach involving educators, healthcare professionals, parents, and the community. Advocacy efforts should focus on:

Increasing Awareness

Raising awareness about the unique presentation of ADHD in girls through campaigns, educational programs, and media can help dispel myths and encourage earlier diagnosis.

Enhancing Training for Educators

Providing specialized training for teachers and school staff on recognizing and addressing ADHD in girls can lead to more timely and accurate identification.

Encouraging Research

Supporting research that explores gender differences in ADHD presentation and outcomes can inform more effective diagnostic tools and interventions.

Promoting Inclusive Policies

Implementing policies that promote mental health awareness and support within educational institutions can create an environment where girls feel safe to seek help.

Fostering Community Support

Building strong support networks, including support groups for girls and families affected by ADHD, can provide essential resources and encouragement.

The early signs of ADHD in girls are often subtle and easily overlooked, leading to significant challenges in childhood that can ripple into adulthood. By understanding the unique manifestations of ADHD in girls, recognizing the profound impact of undiagnosed ADHD on development, education, and self-esteem, and advocating for comprehensive support systems, we can ensure that every girl with ADHD receives the recognition and assistance she deserves. Personal anecdotes and case studies not only humanize these challenges but also serve as powerful reminders of the resilience and potential within each girl facing ADHD. As we move towards a more inclusive and informed society, the early identification and support of ADHD in girls will play a crucial role in empowering them to lead fulfilling and successful lives.

4

Navigating Adulthood: Personal and Professional Life

Transitioning into adulthood presents a myriad of challenges for anyone, but for women with Attention Deficit Hyperactivity Disorder (ADHD), these challenges can be particularly nuanced. ADHD affects various facets of adult life, including career choices, workplace performance, relationships, and daily responsibilities. Understanding these impacts and implementing effective strategies can empower women with ADHD to thrive both personally and professionally.

Understanding the ADHD Adult Landscape

ADHD in adults often manifests differently than in children. While hyperactivity might decrease with age, issues with attention, organization, and time management persist. Women, in particular, may experience internalized symptoms such as chronic disorganization, procrastination, and emotional dysregulation. These symptoms can influence career trajectories, interpersonal relationships, and everyday life in profound ways.

Career Choices: Aligning Strengths with Professional Paths

One of the significant areas where ADHD impacts adulthood is career selection. Women with ADHD may find themselves gravitating toward certain professions that align with their strengths, such as creativity, problem-solving, and the ability to hyperfocus on tasks that interest them. Conversely, they might struggle in careers that demand sustained attention, routine, and extreme organization.

Stories of Transitioning to ADHD-Friendly Careers

Sarah's Journey from Corporate Chaos to Creative Fulfillment

Sarah, a 35-year-old marketing professional, spent over a decade in the corporate sector. Despite her creativity and innovative ideas, she often felt overwhelmed by the rigid structure and constant deadlines. Diagnosed with ADHD in her late twenties, Sarah realized that her struggles stemmed not from a lack of ability but from a mismatch between her ADHD traits and her work environment.

Determined to find a career that suited her strengths, Sarah transitioned into freelance graphic design. This shift allowed her to set her own schedule, choose projects that excited her, and work in a more flexible setting. The change not only improved her job satisfaction but also significantly reduced her stress levels. Sarah's story illustrates how aligning one's career with their natural strengths and ADHD-friendly environments can lead to greater professional fulfillment and personal well-being.

Emily's Path to Entrepreneurship

Emily, a 28-year-old with ADHD, found the conventional office environment stifling. She struggled with micromanagement and rigid schedules, which exacerbated her ADHD symptoms. After consulting with a career coach familiar with ADHD, Emily decided to start her own business as a social media consultant.

As an entrepreneur, Emily could leverage her creativity and enthusiasm for social interactions while minimizing the aspects of work that were challenging for her, such as prolonged periods of monotonous tasks. By creating a business model that played to her strengths and allowed for flexibility, Emily not only built a successful enterprise but also found a sense of autonomy that was previously missing in her corporate job.

Workplace Performance: Challenges and Strategies

ADHD can present significant hurdles in the workplace, affecting performance, relationships with colleagues, and overall job satisfaction. Common challenges include difficulty maintaining focus, poor time management, disorganization, and impulsivity. However, with the right strategies and accommodations, these challenges can be mitigated.

Case Study: Enhancing Productivity through Workplace Accommodations

Jessica's Story: From Overwhelmed to Organized

Jessica, a 32-year-old project manager, was excelling in her role until her ADHD symptoms began to interfere with her performance. She found it challenging to keep track of multiple projects, missed deadlines, and struggled with prioritizing tasks. Recognizing the impact on her career, Jessica sought support from her human resources department.

After disclosing her ADHD diagnosis, Jessica worked with her employer to implement several workplace accommodations:

1. **Flexible Scheduling:** Jessica was allowed to start her day earlier, leveraging her peak productivity hours.
2. **Organizational Tools:** She was provided with project management software and received training on effective time management techniques.
3. **Dedicated Workspace:** Jessica was given a quiet area free from distractions to enhance her focus.

These accommodations led to a remarkable improvement in Jessica's productivity and job satisfaction. She became more organized, met her deadlines consistently, and felt supported by her employer. Jessica's case underscores the importance of workplace accommodations and open communication in enhancing the performance of employees with ADHD.

Relationships: Navigating Personal Connections

ADHD doesn't just impact professional life; it also influences personal relationships. Women with ADHD may face challenges in communication, emotional regulation, and maintaining consistent routines, which can strain friendships, romantic partnerships, and family dynamics.

Anecdote: Managing ADHD in a Long-Term Relationship

Anna and Michael: Building Understanding and Support

Anna, a 40-year-old woman with ADHD, has been in a long-term relationship with her partner, Michael, for over 15 years. In the early years of their relationship, Anna's symptoms often led to misunderstandings. She struggled with forgetfulness, impulsivity, and was frequently late for dates, which frustrated Michael.

Realizing the impact of her ADHD on their relationship, Anna decided to seek therapy. With the help of a therapist specializing in ADHD, both Anna and Michael learned strategies to improve their communication and understanding. They established routines to manage daily tasks, such as setting reminders and using shared calendars. Michael became more patient and educated himself about ADHD, offering support without judgment.

Over time, their relationship strengthened as they developed effective coping mechanisms and built a partnership based on mutual respect and understanding. Anna and Michael's story highlights the importance of open communication, education, and mutual support in managing ADHD within personal relationships.

Daily Responsibilities: Mastering Everyday Tasks

Managing daily responsibilities can be daunting for women with ADHD. Tasks such as household chores, financial management, and personal organization require consistent attention to detail and structure, areas where ADHD can present significant challenges. However, implementing tailored strategies can make daily life more manageable.

Strategies for Managing Daily Responsibilities

1. **Establishing Routines:** Creating consistent daily schedules can help in developing habits that reduce forgetfulness and procrastination.
2. **Using Organizational Tools:** Calendars, to-do lists, and reminder apps can aid in keeping track of tasks and deadlines.
3. **Breaking Tasks into Smaller Steps:** Dividing larger tasks into manageable parts can prevent feeling overwhelmed and increase the likelihood of completion.
4. **Delegating When Possible:** Sharing responsibilities with family members or hiring professional help can alleviate the burden of daily tasks.
5. **Setting Realistic Goals:** Prioritizing tasks and setting achievable goals ensures that essential responsibilities are met without excessive stress.

Strategies for Managing ADHD in Personal and Professional Life

Effectively navigating adulthood with ADHD involves a combination of self-awareness, organizational strategies, and leveraging support systems. Here are several approaches to managing ADHD across various life domains:

1. Time Management Techniques

- **Pomodoro Technique:** Work for 25 minutes, then take a 5-minute break. This cyclical approach can enhance focus and prevent burnout.
- **Time Blocking:** Allocate specific time slots for different tasks throughout the day to ensure balanced attention to various responsibilities.
- **Prioritization Methods:** Use systems like the Eisenhower Matrix to categorize tasks based on urgency and importance.

2. Organizational Strategies

- **Decluttering Workspaces:** Keeping physical and digital workspaces organized can reduce distractions and improve efficiency.
- **Color-Coding Systems:** Utilizing colors to categorize tasks, calendars, or files can enhance visual organization and quick identification of priorities.
- **Consistent Filing Systems:** Implementing uniform filing methods for documents can streamline retrieval and reduce

time spent searching for information.

3. Leveraging Technology

- **Productivity Apps:** Tools like Trello, Asana, or Todoist can assist in task management and project tracking.
- **Reminder Systems:** Setting alarms or notifications on smartphones can help in remembering appointments and deadlines.
- **Note-Taking Applications:** Digital note-taking tools like Evernote or OneNote can capture ideas and important information on the go.

4. Professional Support and Coaching

- **ADHD Coaches:** Specialized coaches can provide personalized strategies and accountability to help manage ADHD symptoms effectively.
- **Therapeutic Interventions:** Cognitive-behavioral therapy (CBT) and other therapeutic approaches can address emotional challenges and develop coping mechanisms.
- **Mentorship Programs:** Connecting with mentors who understand ADHD can offer guidance and support in professional development.

5. Self-Care and Wellness Practices

- **Regular Exercise:** Physical activity can improve focus,

reduce stress, and enhance overall well-being.
- **Balanced Nutrition:** Maintaining a diet rich in nutrients supports brain health and energy levels.
- **Mindfulness and Relaxation Techniques:** Practices such as meditation and yoga can aid in emotional regulation and stress management.

Building a Supportive Environment

Creating a supportive environment, both at home and in the workplace, is crucial for women with ADHD. This involves not only personal strategies but also fostering understanding and collaboration with those around you.

Creating an ADHD-Friendly Home

- **Organized Living Spaces:** Designate specific areas for essentials like keys, wallets, and important documents to minimize daily frustrations.
- **Clear Communication:** Establish open lines of communication with family members to discuss needs and expectations.
- **Supportive Routines:** Develop household routines that accommodate varying energy levels and organizational needs.

Fostering Workplace Support

- **Open Dialogue with Employers:** Discussing ADHD with employers can lead to necessary accommodations, such as flexible work hours or a quieter workspace.
- **Building a Support Network at Work:** Connecting with colleagues who understand ADHD can provide a sense of community and shared strategies.
- **Continuous Professional Development:** Engaging in ongoing learning opportunities can enhance skills and adaptability in the workplace.

Real-Life Success: Thriving with ADHD

Despite the challenges, many women with ADHD have found ways to harness their unique strengths and thrive in both personal and professional realms. Embracing traits such as creativity, resilience, and the ability to think outside the box can turn ADHD from a perceived limitation into a powerful asset.

Anecdote: Leveraging Creativity in the Workplace

Lily's Innovative Solutions

Lily, a 30-year-old software developer with ADHD, often found herself struggling with the repetitive aspects of her job. However, her ADHD also endowed her with a creative approach to problem-solving. Rather than viewing her condition as a hindrance, Lily embraced her ability to think divergently. She proposed and led a project that utilized innovative coding techniques, resulting in a more efficient software solution.

Lily's willingness to leverage her creativity not only advanced her career but also brought fresh perspectives to her team. Her story exemplifies how embracing ADHD-related strengths can lead to professional success and personal satisfaction.

Overcoming Stigmas and Building Confidence

Women with ADHD may face societal stigmas and internalized negative beliefs about their abilities. Overcoming these challenges involves building self-awareness, seeking appropriate support, and fostering a positive self-image.

Developing Self-Awareness

Understanding how ADHD affects various aspects of life is the first step toward effective management. Self-reflection and education about ADHD can empower women to identify their challenges and strengths, setting the foundation for meaningful change.

Seeking Professional Help

Engaging with mental health professionals, such as therapists and ADHD coaches, provides tailored strategies and support. Professional guidance can help in developing coping mechanisms, enhancing organizational skills, and addressing emotional well-being.

Building a Positive Self-Image

Cultivating self-compassion and focusing on personal achievements can reinforce a positive self-image. Celebrating small victories and recognizing progress fosters confidence and motivation to continue navigating adulthood with ADHD.

Embracing Technology and Innovation

In the digital age, numerous tools and technologies are designed to assist individuals with ADHD in managing their symptoms. Embracing these innovations can significantly enhance personal and professional life.

Assistive Technologies

- **Smartphones and Apps:** Leveraging the capabilities of smartphones with apps tailored for task management, reminders, and time tracking can streamline daily responsibilities.
- **Wearable Devices:** Fitness trackers and smartwatches can aid in monitoring physical activity, sleep patterns, and managing time effectively.
- **Voice Assistants:** Utilizing voice-activated assistants like Siri or Alexa can help in setting reminders, making lists, and organizing schedules hands-free.

Financial Management: Strategies for Success

Managing finances can pose unique challenges for women with ADHD, given the tendency towards impulsivity and difficulty in maintaining long-term financial plans. Implementing effective financial management strategies is essential for achieving financial stability and independence.

Budgeting Techniques

- **Automated Savings:** Setting up automatic transfers to savings accounts ensures that saving is consistent and reduces the temptation to spend impulsively.
- **Categorized Budgeting:** Breaking down expenses into categories (e.g., housing, utilities, entertainment) can provide a clear overview of financial obligations and spending habits.
- **Regular Reviews:** Scheduling monthly reviews of financial statements helps in tracking progress and making necessary adjustments.

Tools for Financial Management

- **Budgeting Apps:** Tools like Mint, YNAB (You Need a Budget), and PocketGuard can simplify budgeting, expense tracking, and financial goal setting.
- **Bill Payment Reminders:** Setting up automatic payments and reminders prevents missed payments and associated penalties.
- **Financial Advisors:** Consulting with financial professionals who understand ADHD can offer personalized strategies and support for effective money management.

Setting Realistic Goals and Achieving Them

Goal-setting is a vital aspect of managing ADHD in adulthood. However, it's important to set realistic, achievable goals to maintain motivation and prevent discouragement.

SMART Goals Framework

Using the SMART criteria—Specific, Measurable, Achievable, Relevant, Time-bound—can enhance the effectiveness of goal-setting:

- **Specific:** Clearly define what you want to achieve.
- **Measurable:** Ensure that progress can be tracked.
- **Achievable:** Set realistic goals that are attainable.
- **Relevant:** Align goals with personal values and long-term objectives.
- **Time-bound:** Establish a clear deadline for achieving the goal.

Breaking Down Goals

Dividing larger goals into smaller, manageable tasks makes them less overwhelming and increases the likelihood of success. Celebrating incremental achievements fosters a sense of accomplishment and sustained motivation.

Conclusion: Empowering Women with ADHD to Thrive

Navigating adulthood with ADHD presents unique challenges, but with the right strategies and support, women can transform these challenges into opportunities for growth and success. By understanding how ADHD affects various aspects of life, implementing effective management techniques, and leveraging personal strengths, women with ADHD can create fulfilling personal and professional lives.

Embracing self-awareness, seeking professional support, building a strong support network, and utilizing technology are all integral components of this journey. Moreover, shifting societal perceptions and fostering environments that accommodate and celebrate neurodiversity can pave the way for greater inclusion and empowerment.

As women with ADHD continue to advocate for themselves and others, the narrative around ADHD in adulthood evolves from one of limitation to one of potential and resilience. By embracing their unique strengths and employing tailored strategies, women with ADHD can not only navigate adulthood successfully but also thrive in ways that enrich their lives and the communities around them.

Key Takeaways

- **Self-Awareness:** Understanding how ADHD affects personal and professional life is crucial for effective management.
- **Career Alignment:** Choosing ADHD-friendly careers that leverage strengths can enhance job satisfaction and performance.

- **Workplace Accommodations:** Implementing and advocating for necessary accommodations can mitigate workplace challenges.
- **Relationship Management:** Open communication and mutual understanding are vital for maintaining healthy relationships.
- **Organizational Strategies:** Effective time management, organizational tools, and routines can simplify daily responsibilities.
- **Support Systems:** Building a strong support network, including professional help and community resources, is essential.
- **Embracing Strengths:** Recognizing and leveraging the unique strengths associated with ADHD can lead to personal and professional success.

By integrating these principles into daily life, women with ADHD can overcome obstacles, harness their unique abilities, and create a balanced, fulfilling adulthood.

5

Emotional Well-being and Mental Health

Living with Attention Deficit Hyperactivity Disorder (ADHD) as a woman presents a unique set of emotional challenges. Beyond the well-known symptoms of inattention and hyperactivity, many women grapple with anxiety, depression, and low self-esteem. These emotional burdens can significantly impact daily life, relationships, and overall well-being. This chapter delves into the intricate relationship between ADHD and emotional health, exploring the underlying causes, presenting effective coping mechanisms, and highlighting therapeutic approaches that can pave the way toward emotional resilience and fulfillment.

Understanding the Emotional Landscape of ADHD in Women

ADHD does not exist in isolation from other emotional and psychological states. For women, the interplay between ADHD and emotions is often intensified by societal expectations, gender norms, and internal pressures. Unlike their male counterparts, women with ADHD may internalize their struggles more, leading to a higher incidence of anxiety and depression.

1. Anxiety and ADHD

Anxiety frequently coexists with ADHD, creating a complex emotional landscape. The constant battle to stay organized, meet deadlines, and maintain relationships can lead to chronic stress. Women with ADHD often feel overwhelmed by the demands of daily life, which exacerbates anxiety symptoms. The fear of failure and the anticipation of not meeting expectations can be paralyzing, making it difficult to navigate both personal and professional realms.

2. Depression and ADHD

Depression is another common companion to ADHD in women. Persistent feelings of inadequacy, frustration, and hopelessness can stem from the continuous struggle to manage ADHD symptoms. When efforts to stay organized or complete tasks consistently fall short, it can lead to a pervasive sense of failure, fostering depressive thoughts. Additionally, hormonal fluctuations, such as those experienced during menstrual cycles, can further intensify depressive symptoms, creating a challenging emotional cycle.

3. Low Self-esteem

Low self-esteem is a pervasive issue for many women with ADHD. Societal standards often dictate that women should be inherently organized, emotionally stable, and adept at multitasking. When ADHD disrupts these expectations, women may internalize a negative self-image, viewing themselves as incapable or inadequate. This diminished self-worth can hinder personal growth, career advancement, and the ability to form healthy relationships.

The Root Causes of Emotional Challenges
    Understanding why women with ADHD experience height-
ened emotional challenges requires a multifaceted approach,
considering both biological and societal factors.

1. Neurobiological Factors

Research indicates that ADHD is associated with dysregulation in brain regions responsible for executive function, emotional regulation, and impulse control. Neurotransmitter imbalances, particularly involving dopamine and norepinephrine,
play a crucial role in both ADHD and mood disorders. These
biological underpinnings can predispose women with ADHD to
experience heightened emotional reactivity and susceptibility
to anxiety and depression.

2. Hormonal Influences

Hormonal fluctuations inherent in women's lives, such
as those occurring during menstrual cycles, pregnancy, and
menopause, can significantly impact ADHD symptoms and
emotional health. Estrogen and progesterone levels affect
neurotransmitter activity, influencing mood and cognitive
function. For instance, premenstrual dysphoric disorder
(PMDD) shares symptoms with ADHD-related emotional
dysregulation, exacerbating anxiety and depressive tendencies
during certain phases of the menstrual cycle.

3. Societal and Cultural Expectations

Societal norms often place a premium on women's ability to
juggle multiple roles effortlessly—being a competent profes-

sional, a nurturing parent, a caring partner, and a responsible household manager. Women with ADHD, who may struggle with time management, organizational skills, and emotional regulation, find these expectations particularly daunting. The pressure to conform to these standards can lead to chronic stress, anxiety, and a diminished sense of self-worth.

4. Underdiagnosis and Misdiagnosis

ADHD in women is frequently underdiagnosed or misdiagnosed, often being mistaken for anxiety, depression, or personality disorders. This misdiagnosis means that the core issues related to ADHD remain unaddressed, perpetuating emotional distress. Without appropriate diagnosis and treatment, women continue to grapple with unmanaged symptoms, leading to worsening mental health over time.

Coping Mechanisms for Emotional Well-being

Despite the challenges, there are effective strategies and coping mechanisms that women with ADHD can employ to enhance their emotional well-being. These strategies span lifestyle adjustments, therapeutic interventions, and self-care practices.

1. Mindfulness and Meditation

Mindfulness practices can be particularly beneficial for managing the emotional turbulence associated with ADHD. By fostering present-moment awareness, mindfulness helps reduce anxiety by preventing the mind from dwelling on past failures or future uncertainties. Regular meditation can enhance emotional regulation, increase resilience to stress, and improve concentration.

Practical Tip: Start with short, guided meditation sessions using apps like Headspace or Calm. Gradually increase the duration as you become more comfortable with the practice.

2. Cognitive-Behavioral Techniques

Cognitive-behavioral techniques can help women with ADHD challenge and reframe negative thought patterns. By identifying cognitive distortions—such as all-or-nothing thinking or catastrophizing—and replacing them with more balanced perspectives, individuals can mitigate feelings of anxiety and depression.

Practical Tip: Keep a thought journal to track negative thoughts and systematically evaluate their validity. Work with a therapist to develop healthier cognitive patterns.

3. Physical Activity and Exercise

Regular physical activity has been shown to improve mood, reduce anxiety, and enhance cognitive function. Exercise stimulates the release of endorphins, which are natural mood lifters, and can also aid in the regulation of neurotransmitters associated with ADHD.

Practical Tip: Incorporate activities you enjoy, whether it's yoga, dancing, running, or hiking. Aim for at least 30 minutes of moderate exercise most days of the week.

4. Structured Routine and Organization

Establishing a structured daily routine can alleviate the chaos that often exacerbates emotional distress. Predictable schedules reduce uncertainty, helping to manage anxiety and foster a sense of control.

Practical Tip: Use planners, calendars, or digital apps to organize your day. Break tasks into smaller, manageable steps and prioritize them to prevent feeling overwhelmed.

5. Social Support Networks

Building and maintaining strong social support networks can provide emotional sustenance and practical assistance. Sharing experiences with others who understand can reduce feelings of isolation and foster a sense of belonging.

Practical Tip: Join ADHD support groups, both in-person and online. Engage with friends and family members who offer encouragement and understanding.

6. Self-Compassion and Acceptance

Cultivating self-compassion involves treating oneself with kindness and understanding, especially during moments of struggle. Accepting ADHD as a part of one's identity rather than viewing it solely as a limitation can enhance self-esteem and emotional resilience.

Practical Tip: Practice self-affirmations and challenge self-critical thoughts. Remind yourself of your strengths and accomplishments regularly.

Therapeutic Approaches for Emotional Health

Professional therapeutic interventions can play a crucial role in managing the emotional challenges associated with ADHD. Below are some evidence-based therapies that have proven effective for women with ADHD.

1. Cognitive-Behavioral Therapy (CBT)

CBT is a structured, goal-oriented therapy that focuses on identifying and modifying negative thought patterns and behaviors. For women with ADHD, CBT can address co-occurring anxiety and depression by teaching coping strategies and fostering healthier cognitive frameworks.

Case Study: Sarah's Journey with CBT

Sarah, a 35-year-old marketing executive, struggled with undiagnosed ADHD for most of her adult life. Her symptoms included chronic procrastination, disorganization, and persistent anxiety about her professional performance. After years of feeling overwhelmed and unfulfilled, Sarah sought therapy.

Through CBT, Sarah learned to identify her negative self-talk, such as "I'm never going to get anything right" and "I can't handle my responsibilities." Her therapist helped her challenge these thoughts by examining the evidence and considering more balanced perspectives. Additionally, Sarah developed practical skills for time management and organization, which reduced her anxiety by providing a clearer structure to her day.

Over six months of CBT, Sarah experienced significant improvements in her mood and productivity. She reported feeling more confident in her abilities and less overwhelmed by her responsibilities. CBT empowered Sarah to manage both her ADHD symptoms and the associated emotional challenges, leading to a more balanced and fulfilling life.

2. Dialectical Behavior Therapy (DBT)

DBT combines cognitive-behavioral techniques with mindfulness practices. It emphasizes the development of skills in emotional regulation, distress tolerance, interpersonal effectiveness, and mindfulness. For women with ADHD, DBT can be particularly effective in managing intense emotions and improving relational dynamics.

3. Mindfulness-Based Cognitive Therapy (MBCT)

MBCT integrates mindfulness practices with cognitive therapy techniques. It aims to prevent the relapse of depression by fostering greater awareness and acceptance of one's thoughts and feelings. This approach can help women with ADHD break the cycle of rumination and emotional dysregulation.

4. Narrative Therapy

Narrative therapy involves re-authoring one's life story to highlight strengths and resilience rather than focusing solely on challenges. For women with ADHD, narrative therapy can help redefine their identity beyond their symptoms, promoting a more positive self-concept and emotional well-being.

5. Medication Management

While not a therapy per se, medication can significantly impact emotional health by managing ADHD symptoms. Stimulant and non-stimulant medications can improve focus, reduce impulsivity, and enhance emotional regulation, thereby alleviating anxiety and depressive symptoms. It is essential to work closely with a healthcare provider to find the most effective and tolerable medication regimen.

Personal Narratives: Overcoming Emotional Hurdles

Hearing from women who have navigated the emotional labyrinth of ADHD can provide both inspiration and practical insights. These personal stories illuminate the diverse ways ADHD intersects with emotional well-being and offer hope for those seeking to overcome similar challenges.

Anecdote 1: Emma's Battle with Anxiety

Emma, a 29-year-old graphic designer, always felt different from her peers. While she excelled in creative tasks, she struggled with deadlines, organization, and maintaining focus. Her undiagnosed ADHD led to chronic anxiety, as she constantly feared letting others down.

After years of frustration, Emma sought therapy and received her ADHD diagnosis. With the help of her therapist, she learned mindfulness techniques to manage her anxiety and developed organizational strategies tailored to her needs. Emma also joined a support group, where she connected with other women facing similar challenges. These steps not only reduced her anxiety but also boosted her self-esteem, enabling her to thrive in her career and personal life.

Anecdote 2: Maya's Journey Through Depression

Maya, a 42-year-old mother of two, battled depression that masked her ADHD symptoms. She felt perpetually exhausted, overwhelmed by household responsibilities, and disconnected from her ambitions. Maya's depression was compounded by her inability to manage ADHD-related tasks, creating a toxic cycle of self-criticism and hopelessness.

Upon diagnosing her ADHD, Maya began cognitive-behavioral therapy focusing on both her ADHD and depressive symptoms. She learned to set realistic goals, prioritize tasks, and practice self-compassion. Mindfulness meditation became a daily ritual, helping her stay grounded amidst the chaos of motherhood. Over time, Maya's depression lifted, and she rediscovered her sense of purpose and joy.

Building Emotional Resilience: Strategies for Long-term Well-being

Emotional resilience—the ability to adapt and thrive despite adversity—is crucial for women with ADHD. Developing resilience involves cultivating a positive mindset, fostering supportive relationships, and maintaining healthy habits.

1. Cultivating a Positive Mindset

Adopting a growth mindset—the belief that abilities and intelligence can be developed through dedication and hard work—can transform how women with ADHD perceive their challenges. Viewing setbacks as opportunities for learning rather than as reflections of inadequacy fosters resilience and persistence.

Practical Exercise: Reflect on past challenges and identify what you learned from them. Replace negative narratives with positive affirmations that highlight your growth and strengths.

2. Building a Supportive Community

Surrounding oneself with understanding and supportive individuals is essential for emotional health. Friends, family, support groups, and mental health professionals can provide encouragement, accountability, and practical assistance.

Practical Tip: Actively seek out communities—both in-person and online—that offer support for women with ADHD. Engage in meaningful conversations and share your experiences to build a network of allies.

3. Prioritizing Self-Care

Self-care is not a luxury but a necessity for maintaining emotional well-being. Incorporating regular self-care activities—such as hobbies, relaxation, exercise, and adequate sleep—can replenish emotional reserves and reduce stress.

Practical Tip: Schedule self-care into your daily routine as you would any other important activity. Identify activities that bring you joy and relaxation, and make them a non-negotiable part of your day.

4. Setting Realistic Goals

Setting attainable goals provides a sense of direction and accomplishment. Breaking larger objectives into smaller, manageable tasks can prevent feeling overwhelmed and foster a sense of progress.

Practical Tip: Use SMART goals—specific, measurable, achievable, relevant, and time-bound—to structure your objectives. Regularly review and adjust your goals to stay aligned with your evolving priorities.

5. Embracing Flexibility and Adaptability

Life is inherently unpredictable, and the ability to adapt to changing circumstances is a key component of emotional resilience. Embracing flexibility allows women with ADHD to navigate life's ups and downs with greater ease.

Practical Tip: Practice accepting that not everything will go according to plan. Develop contingency plans and remain open to alternative solutions when faced with unexpected challenges.

The Role of Self-Compassion in Emotional Well-being

Self-compassion involves treating oneself with the same kindness and understanding that one would offer to a friend in distress. For women with ADHD, self-compassion can counteract the harsh self-criticism that often accompanies emotional struggles.

1. The Three Components of Self-Compassion

According to Dr. Kristin Neff, self-compassion comprises three core components:

- **Self-Kindness:** Being gentle and understanding with oneself rather than harshly critical.
- **Common Humanity:** Recognizing that suffering and personal inadequacy are part of the shared human experience.
- **Mindfulness:** Maintaining a balanced awareness of one's emotions without over-identifying with them.

2. Practicing Self-Compassion

Cultivating self-compassion involves intentional practices that reinforce kindness, connectedness, and mindful awareness.

Practical Exercises:

- **Self-Compassion Break:** When experiencing emotional distress, take a moment to place a hand over your heart, acknowledge your suffering ("This is a moment of suffering"), remind yourself of shared humanity ("Many people struggle with this"), and offer yourself kind words ("May I be kind to myself in this moment").
- **Journaling:** Regularly write about your experiences with self-compassion. Reflect on moments when you were hard on yourself and practice reframing those thoughts with greater kindness.
- **Affirmations:** Develop a set of affirming statements that reinforce your worth and capabilities. Repeat these affirmations daily to build a compassionate inner narrative.

3. Overcoming Barriers to Self-Compassion

Women with ADHD may face internal barriers to self-compassion, such as entrenched negative self-beliefs and perfectionism. Addressing these barriers requires persistent effort and, often, professional guidance.

Practical Tip: Work with a therapist to identify and challenge self-critical patterns. Engage in activities that promote self-compassion, such as mindfulness meditation and compassionate imagery exercises.

Navigating the Intersection of ADHD and Emotional Health: A Holistic Approach

Addressing emotional well-being in women with ADHD necessitates a holistic approach that integrates various strategies and supports. By combining lifestyle adjustments, therapeutic interventions, and self-care practices, women can cultivate emotional resilience and achieve a balanced, fulfilling life.

1. Integrated Treatment Plans

Effective management of ADHD and its emotional repercussions often requires an integrated treatment plan that addresses both the neurological and psychological aspects of the disorder. Collaboration between healthcare providers, therapists, and support networks ensures a comprehensive approach tailored to individual needs.

2. Personalized Strategies

What works for one person may not work for another. Personalizing coping strategies and therapeutic interventions is crucial for effective emotional management. This personalization involves understanding one's unique triggers, strengths, and preferences.

Practical Tip: Engage in self-reflection to identify which strategies resonate most with you. Be open to experimenting with different approaches to discover what best supports your emotional well-being.

3. Continuous Learning and Adaptation

Emotional well-being is an ongoing journey, not a destination. Continuously learning about ADHD, staying informed about new treatment modalities, and adapting strategies as circumstances change are essential for sustained emotional health.

Practical Tip: Stay engaged with ADHD communities, attend workshops, and seek out new resources to expand your knowledge and adapt to evolving needs.

Moving Forward: Embracing Emotional Wellness

Embracing emotional wellness as a woman with ADHD involves acknowledging the challenges, celebrating the strengths, and committing to continuous growth. By prioritizing emotional health, women with ADHD can break free from the chains of anxiety, depression, and low self-esteem, paving the way for a life marked by resilience, joy, and fulfillment.

1. Celebrating Strengths and Achievements

Women with ADHD often possess unique strengths such as creativity, empathy, and the ability to think outside the box. Recognizing and celebrating these strengths can enhance self-esteem and provide a foundation for emotional well-being.

Practical Tip: Maintain a gratitude journal where you regularly note your strengths and achievements, no matter how small.

Reflecting on these can reinforce a positive self-image.

2. Setting Boundaries and Prioritizing Needs

Setting healthy boundaries is crucial for protecting emotional well-being. By clearly defining personal limits and prioritizing one's needs, women with ADHD can prevent burnout and foster healthier relationships.

Practical Tip: Learn to say no when necessary and communicate your boundaries clearly to others. Prioritize activities and commitments that align with your well-being.

3. Seeking Professional Help When Needed

Professional support can provide invaluable assistance in managing the emotional challenges of ADHD. Therapists, counselors, and coaches specialized in ADHD can offer tailored guidance and support.

Practical Tip: Don't hesitate to seek professional help if you're struggling with emotional challenges. Regular check-ins with a mental health professional can provide ongoing support and strategies.

4. Embracing a Growth Mindset

Adopting a growth mindset—believing that abilities and intelligence can be developed through effort and perseverance—can transform how women with ADHD perceive their challenges and potential.

Practical Tip: Reframe setbacks as opportunities for growth and learning. Embrace challenges as chances to develop new skills and strengths.

Emotional well-being is a cornerstone of a fulfilling life, and for women with ADHD, navigating this terrain requires a nuanced understanding and a multifaceted approach. By acknowledging the unique emotional challenges associated with ADHD, embracing effective coping mechanisms, and seeking supportive therapeutic interventions, women can cultivate resilience and achieve emotional harmony. Personal narratives and case studies exemplify the transformative power of these strategies, offering hope and practical guidance for those on their journey toward emotional well-being.

As you continue to explore and implement the strategies discussed in this chapter, remember that the path to emotional wellness is a continuous journey. Celebrate your progress, seek support when needed, and remain compassionate with yourself. Embracing your emotional well-being is not only a step toward managing ADHD but also a profound investment in your overall happiness and fulfillment.

6

Relationships and Social Dynamics

Introduction

For many women with Attention Deficit Hyperactivity Disorder (ADHD), navigating relationships and social dynamics can be both rewarding and challenging. ADHD symptoms—such as impulsivity, distractibility, and emotional volatility—can significantly impact friendships, romantic partnerships, and family interactions. Understanding these effects and developing effective strategies is crucial for fostering healthy, supportive, and enduring relationships. This chapter delves into the complexities of ADHD in various relational contexts, offering guidance on communication, empathy, and mutual support to build and maintain meaningful connections.

ADHD in Friendships

Friendships are a fundamental aspect of social life, providing emotional support, companionship, and a sense of belonging. However, ADHD can influence these relationships in several ways:

1. **Forgetfulness and Reliability Issues:** Women with ADHD may struggle with remembering plans, deadlines, or important dates, leading friends to perceive them as unreliable or disinterested. Forgetting birthdays or failing to show up for scheduled meet-ups can strain friendships.

2. **Impulsivity and Social Sensitivity:** Impulsive behaviors, such as interrupting conversations or making hasty decisions, can disrupt the flow of interactions. Additionally, heightened emotional sensitivity can lead to misunderstandings or overreactions during social exchanges.

3. **Difficulty Maintaining Focus:** Staying engaged during conversations or group activities can be challenging, causing friends to feel dismissed or undervalued.

Strategies for Building and Maintaining Friendships:

- **Open Communication:** Being honest about ADHD can help friends understand certain behaviors. Explaining that forgetfulness or distractibility is not a lack of care can mitigate misunderstandings.

- **Use of Reminders:** Leveraging tools like phone alarms, calendars, and reminder apps can help manage forgetfulness. Setting up regular catch-ups or using scheduling apps can ensure consistent interaction.

- **Active Listening Techniques:** Practicing mindfulness and active listening can improve focus during conversations. Techniques such as repeating back what was heard or asking clarifying questions can enhance engagement.

- **Setting Realistic Expectations:** Recognizing personal limits and communicating these can prevent overcommitment and reduce stress within friendships. It's important to

73

balance social activities with personal needs.

ADHD in Romantic Relationships

Romantic relationships often demand a higher level of emotional intimacy and mutual support, making them particularly susceptible to the challenges posed by ADHD. The intricacies of romantic partnerships mean that ADHD-related behaviors can have a profound impact on the relationship's dynamics.

Common Challenges:

1. **Communication Breakdowns:** Misunderstandings may arise from impulsive remarks, inattentiveness, or misinterpretation of intentions. These communication gaps can lead to frustration and resentment.
2. **Emotional Regulation:** Women with ADHD might experience heightened emotional responses, leading to mood swings or increased sensitivity during conflicts.
3. **Shared Responsibilities:** Managing household duties, financial tasks, and parenting responsibilities can become contentious if ADHD symptoms interfere with consistent participation.
4. **Intimacy and Connection:** Maintaining emotional and physical intimacy requires sustained attention and emotional availability, which can be challenging amidst ADHD symptoms like distractibility or fatigue.

Anecdote: Managing ADHD in a Long-Term Relationship

Take the example of Sarah and Michael, a couple married for ten years. Sarah was diagnosed with ADHD in her late twenties, after years of her symptoms being misunderstood by those around her. Before her diagnosis, Sarah often felt she was falling short in her marriage—forgetting important dates, losing track of shared responsibilities, and feeling emotionally volatile. Michael, initially unaware of ADHD, struggled to understand why Sarah seemed disengaged or unreliable at times.

Upon her diagnosis, Sarah and Michael began attending couples therapy to better understand ADHD's role in their relationship. They learned to communicate more effectively, with Sarah setting up reminders for important tasks and Michael becoming more patient and supportive. Through open dialogue and mutual effort, they developed strategies to strengthen their relationship, transforming previously frustrating challenges into opportunities for growth and deeper connection.

Strategies for Enhancing Romantic Relationships:

- **Educate Each Other:** Both partners should educate themselves about ADHD to foster understanding and empathy. This shared knowledge can bridge gaps in perception and reduce blame.
- **Structured Communication:** Implementing regular check-ins or scheduled conversations can ensure that both partners have designated times to discuss concerns and needs without the pressure of spontaneous dialogue.
- **Divide Responsibilities Fairly:** Clearly delineating household tasks and responsibilities can prevent overwhelm. Using tools like chore charts or task management apps can help distribute duties more evenly.
- **Emotional Support:** Cultivating emotional intelligence and practicing empathy can strengthen the emotional bond.

Partners should strive to support each other's emotional well-being actively.

Family Dynamics

ADHD doesn't exist in isolation; it influences and is influenced by family dynamics. Whether it's in the roles parents, siblings, or extended family play, ADHD can alter the traditional patterns of interaction and support within a family unit.

Impact on Family Roles:

1. **Parenting:** Parents with ADHD might find it challenging to maintain consistent parenting practices, manage household routines, or keep up with their children's academic and extracurricular activities. This inconsistency can affect children's behavior, academic performance, and emotional health.
2. **Sibling Relationships:** Siblings may experience shifts in dynamics as a family member with ADHD demands more attention or exhibits behaviors that disrupt the usual harmony. This can lead to feelings of neglect or resentment among siblings.
3. **Spousal Relationships:** Similar to romantic partnerships, spousal relationships can face strains if ADHD symptoms interfere with mutual support, communication, and shared responsibilities.

Case Study: Family Strategies to Support a Member with ADHD

Consider the Thompson family, where Laura, a mother of two, was diagnosed with ADHD after years of unnoticed symptoms. Before her diagnosis, Laura struggled to manage household tasks, leading to frequent arguments with her husband, Tom, and feelings of inadequacy. Her children, ages eight and ten, began exhibiting behavioral issues linked to the inconsiderate atmosphere at home.

After Laura's diagnosis, the family sought the help of a family therapist specializing in ADHD. They implemented several strategies:

- **Clear Communication:** The family established open lines of communication, allowing Laura to express her frustrations and receive support without judgment.
- **Structured Routines:** Implementing a daily routine helped manage household tasks more effectively. Visual schedules and checklists made it easier for Laura to stay on track.
- **Delegated Responsibilities:** Tasks were delegated based on each family member's strengths, reducing the burden on Laura and promoting a sense of teamwork.
- **Emotional Support:** The family prioritized emotional support, ensuring that Laura and the children could express their feelings and receive validation.

Over time, these strategies led to improved household harmony, better academic performance from the children, and a stronger familial bond. Laura felt more competent and supported, reducing her stress and enhancing her ability to manage ADHD symptoms.

Strategies for Improving Family Dynamics:

- **Seek Professional Guidance:** Family therapy can provide a neutral space to address conflicts and develop effective strategies tailored to the family's unique needs.

· **Establish Routines and Structure:** Consistent schedules and clear expectations can help mitigate the unpredictability that ADHD symptoms may introduce into family life.
· **Promote Open Communication:** Encouraging all family members to express their thoughts and feelings can foster understanding and reduce tensions.
· **Support Each Other:** Recognizing that ADHD affects everyone differently, family members should strive to support one another's strengths and challenges.

Communication Strategies

Effective communication is the cornerstone of any healthy relationship, yet ADHD can complicate interactions in several ways. Developing robust communication techniques is essential for women with ADHD and their loved ones to foster understanding and minimize conflicts.

Active Listening:

Active listening involves fully concentrating on the speaker, understanding their message, and responding thoughtfully. For someone with ADHD, practicing active listening can help mitigate distractibility and improve the quality of interactions.

· **Techniques:**
· Maintain eye contact.
· Avoid interrupting.
· Paraphrase what the other person said to ensure understanding.

Expressing Needs Clearly:

Women with ADHD often have specific needs related to their condition. Clearly articulating these needs to friends and partners can facilitate better support and accommodations.

- **Techniques:**
- Use "I" statements to express feelings (e.g., "I feel overwhelmed when...").
- Be specific about what support is needed (e.g., reminders for appointments).

Setting Boundaries:
Healthy boundaries are crucial in maintaining balanced relationships and preventing burnout.

- **Techniques:**
- Identify personal limits.
- Communicate boundaries respectfully.
- Be consistent in enforcing boundaries.

Non-Verbal Communication:
Understanding and utilizing non-verbal cues can enhance relationships and reduce misunderstandings.

- **Techniques:**
- Pay attention to body language and facial expressions.
- Use appropriate gestures to convey messages.
- Ensure congruence between verbal and non-verbal messages.

Building Supportive Relationships
Supportive relationships provide the emotional and practical

assistance necessary for managing ADHD effectively. Building a network of understanding and empathetic individuals can significantly enhance the quality of life for women with ADHD.

Finding Understanding Partners:

Surrounding oneself with partners, friends, and family members who understand ADHD and are willing to offer support is invaluable. These individuals can provide empathy, patience, and practical assistance in navigating daily challenges.

Support Groups and Communities:

Joining ADHD support groups or online communities can offer a sense of belonging and shared experience. These groups provide a platform to exchange strategies, share successes and setbacks, and receive encouragement.

Seeking Therapy or Counseling:

Professional counseling can help individuals with ADHD and their loved ones develop effective coping mechanisms and communication strategies. Therapists can offer personalized guidance and support tailored to specific relational dynamics.

Managing Conflict

Conflict is a natural part of any relationship, but ADHD can intensify disagreements due to communication breakdowns, impulsivity, and emotional volatility. Developing effective conflict resolution strategies is essential for maintaining healthy relationships.

Identifying Triggers:

Understanding the specific triggers that lead to conflicts can help in addressing the root causes. Common triggers might include unmet expectations, miscommunications, or stress from external factors.

Conflict Resolution Techniques:

1. **Stay Calm:** Taking deep breaths and pausing before responding can prevent impulsive reactions.
2. **Focus on Solutions:** Rather than dwelling on the problem, shift the conversation towards finding practical solutions.
3. **Empathize:** Attempt to understand the other person's perspective and validate their feelings.
4. **Agree to Disagree:** Recognize that not all conflicts can be resolved immediately and that some differences are acceptable.

Self-Advocacy in Relationships

Self-advocacy involves understanding and expressing one's own needs and rights within relationships. For women with ADHD, effective self-advocacy can lead to more balanced and supportive interactions.

Understanding Personal Needs:

Identifying how ADHD affects personal life and relationships is the first step in advocating for necessary changes or accommodations.

Communicating About ADHD:

Discussing ADHD openly with partners and friends can foster understanding and reduce stigma. Education about the condition can help loved ones offer appropriate support.

Setting Goals:

Creating clear, achievable goals related to relationship management can provide direction and motivation. These goals might include improving communication skills, managing time more effectively, or seeking joint counseling.

Encouraging Mutual Understanding

Mutual understanding between individuals with ADHD and their loved ones is crucial for fostering empathy and reducing conflicts. Encouraging this understanding involves education, empathy, and consistent effort from both parties.

Educating Loved Ones:

Providing resources about ADHD, such as books, articles, or workshops, can help partners and friends gain a deeper insight into the condition.

Building Empathy:

Encouraging empathy involves promoting active listening and perspective-taking. Partners and friends should strive to understand the emotional experiences of women with ADHD.

Reducing Stigma:

Challenging societal misconceptions and stigmas surrounding ADHD can foster a more accepting and supportive environment within personal relationships.

ADHD significantly influences relationships and social interactions, presenting unique challenges that women must navigate in their friendships, romantic partnerships, and family dynamics. However, with self-awareness, effective communication, and supportive strategies, it is entirely possible to cultivate and maintain healthy, fulfilling relationships. By embracing understanding, empathy, and proactive management of ADHD symptoms, women can build strong relational foundations that support their well-being and personal growth. Remember, the journey towards harmonious relationships is ongoing, requiring patience, effort, and mutual respect from all parties involved.

Final Thoughts

Relationships are a vital component of well-being, and ADHD should not be seen as a barrier but rather as a unique aspect of one's personality that, with the right strategies and support, can coexist harmoniously within social dynamics. Embracing the strengths that come with ADHD—such as creativity, spontaneity, and resilience—can further enrich relationships, turning potential challenges into opportunities for deeper connection and mutual growth.

References:

- Barkley, R. A. (2014). *Attention-Deficit Hyperactivity Disorder: A Handbook for Diagnosis and Treatment.* Guilford Publications.
- Solanto, M. V. (2011). *Cognitive-Behavioral Therapy for Adult ADHD: An Integrative Psychosocial and Medical Approach.* Guilford Press.
- Young, S. (2015). *ADHD and Women: Love, Relationships and Emotional Life.* New Harbinger Publications.

7

Parenting with ADHD: Balancing Personal Needs and Childcare

Parenting is a rewarding yet demanding journey, requiring patience, organization, and emotional resilience. For women with Attention Deficit Hyperactivity Disorder (ADHD), these demands can be compounded by unique challenges that affect both personal well-being and the dynamics of family life. This chapter delves into the intricate balance of managing ADHD while nurturing children, offering practical strategies and real-life examples to empower mothers in their parenting roles.

Understanding the Dual Role: Mother and Individual with ADHD
Parenting involves wearing multiple hats: caregiver, teacher, disciplinarian, and emotional supporter. For women with ADHD, these roles can sometimes clash with the personal challenges posed by the disorder, such as difficulties with attention, executive functioning, and emotional regulation. Recognizing the interplay between personal ADHD symptoms and parenting responsibilities is the first step toward creating a harmonious family environment.

Key Challenges:

- **Executive Dysfunction:** Struggling with planning, organizing, and following through on tasks can make daily routines and household management overwhelming.
- **Emotional Regulation:** ADHD often comes with heightened emotional responses, which can impact interactions with children and lead to misunderstandings or conflicts.
- **Time Management:** Keeping track of schedules, appointments, and deadlines can be particularly challenging, leading to missed activities or a sense of constant chaos.
- **Impulsivity:** Making quick decisions without thorough consideration can affect parenting choices and consistency in discipline.

Implementing ADHD-Friendly Routines: A Story of Structure and Success

Creating structured routines is paramount for families navigating ADHD. Routines provide predictability, reduce stress, and foster a sense of security for children. However, establishing and maintaining these routines can be daunting for parents with ADHD.

Anecdote: Sarah's ADHD-Friendly Morning Routine

Sarah, a 35-year-old mother of two, was constantly battling morning chaos. Mornings were a whirlwind of forgotten school lunches, missed appointments, and last-minute scrambles to get everyone out the door on time. Her ADHD symptoms—particularly difficulty with organization and time management—made mornings incredibly stressful.

Determined to create a more peaceful start to her day, Sarah implemented the following ADHD-friendly strategies:

1. **Visual Schedules:** Sarah created a large, colorful calendar placed in the kitchen, outlining morning tasks for each family member. Pictures and icons were used to represent activities (e.g., a drawing of a sandwich for lunch preparation), making it easier for her younger child to follow.
2. **Night Before Preparation:** To minimize morning chaos, Sarah began preparing the night before. Clothes were laid out, backpacks were packed, and breakfast items were set on the table. This reduced the number of tasks to be tackled in the morning, alleviating last-minute stress.
3. **Timers and Alarms:** Using timers for each task helped Sarah stay on track. An alarm signaling "time to wake up," "time to brush teeth," and "time to leave the house" kept the family moving smoothly from one activity to the next without the need for constant supervision.
4. **Dedicated Spaces:** Each family member had a designated spot for their belongings. Hooks for coats, containers for school supplies, and specific areas for keys and shoes ensured that items were easy to find, reducing the time spent searching for lost items.

Within a few weeks, Sarah noticed significant improvements. Mornings became more predictable, and the reduced stress allowed her to focus better on the day's tasks. Additionally, her children thrived in the structured environment, feeling more secure and independent.

Strategies for Effective Parenting with ADHD

Balancing the demands of parenting while managing ADHD symptoms requires intentional strategies that cater to both personal needs and family dynamics. Here are several approaches that can make this balance achievable:

- Prioritize Self-Care:
- Why It Matters: Managing ADHD effectively requires energy and mental clarity. Neglecting self-care can exacerbate symptoms and reduce the capacity to handle parenting challenges.
- How to Implement: Schedule regular self-care activities, such as exercise, meditation, or hobbies. Even small, consistent practices can significantly improve overall well-being.

- Utilize Technology and Tools:
- Why It Matters: Technology can compensate for memory lapses and organizational challenges inherent to ADHD.
- How to Implement: Use smartphone apps for reminders, calendars for scheduling, and organizational tools like to-do lists or bullet journals. Voice-activated assistants (e.g., Amazon Alexa, Google Assistant) can also help manage daily tasks and reminders.

- Delegate and Share Responsibilities:
- Why It Matters: Attempting to handle all responsibilities alone can lead to burnout and increased ADHD symptoms.

- How to Implement: Share household tasks with a partner or older children. Create a family chore chart to distribute responsibilities evenly, ensuring that no single individual is overwhelmed.

- Set Realistic Expectations:
- Why It Matters: Perfectionism and high self-expectations can lead to frustration and decreased self-esteem when they remain unmet.
- How to Implement: Acknowledge limitations and set achievable goals. Celebrate small victories and progress rather than striving for perfection in every task.

- Establish Clear Communication:
- Why It Matters: ADHD can sometimes lead to misunderstandings or inconsistent communication, affecting family relationships.
- How to Implement: Practice active listening and clear, concise communication with family members. Regular family meetings can provide a platform to discuss schedules, expectations, and any issues that arise.

- Create Organizational Systems:
- Why It Matters: Organization is a common struggle for individuals with ADHD, impacting the ability to maintain a

tidy and functional household.

- How to Implement: Implement simple organization systems such as labeled storage bins, designated areas for frequently used items, and regular decluttering sessions. Visual aids like checklists and charts can also help keep the household running smoothly.

Maintaining Household Organization

A well-organized home can significantly reduce stress and create a more conducive environment for both parenting and managing ADHD. Here are some strategies to maintain household organization:

- **Declutter Regularly:**
- **Purpose:** Reduces visual distractions and makes it easier to find essential items.
- **Method:** Set aside time each week to declutter specific areas. Use the "one in, one out" rule to prevent accumulation of unnecessary items.

- **Designate Specific Areas for Items:**
- **Purpose:** Ensures that everyone knows where things belong, making tidying up a straightforward task.
- **Method:** Assign specific spots for common items like keys, wallets, and school supplies. Use labels to reinforce these designated areas.

- **Create a Command Center:**
- **Purpose:** Centralizes important information and items, making it easier to manage household activities.
- **Method:** Set up a command center in a common area with a calendar, whiteboard, mail organizer, and hooks for keys. This serves as a hub for daily schedules and reminders.

- **Implement Daily Cleaning Habits:**
- **Purpose:** Prevents mess from becoming overwhelming and maintains a tidy environment.
- **Method:** Incorporate small cleaning tasks into the daily routine, such as making beds, wiping down surfaces, and sorting mail.

- **Use Storage Solutions:**
- **Purpose:** Keeps items organized and out of sight, reducing clutter and promoting order.
- **Method:** Invest in storage bins, drawer dividers, and shelving units. Ensure that storage solutions are accessible to all family members.

Managing Personal ADHD Symptoms While Caring for Children

Balancing personal ADHD management with parenting responsibilities requires a multifaceted approach that addresses both aspects simultaneously. Here are strategies to effectively manage personal ADHD symptoms while fulfilling parenting duties:

- **Consistent Medication and Treatment Plans:**
- **Purpose:** Effective management of ADHD symptoms can improve focus, organization, and emotional regulation.
- **Method:** Adhere to prescribed medication schedules and regularly consult with healthcare providers to adjust treatments as necessary.

- **Developing Time Management Skills:**
- **Purpose:** Enhances the ability to keep track of multiple responsibilities and reduces the likelihood of missing important tasks.
- **Method:** Use planners, digital calendars, and alarms to organize daily activities. Break tasks into smaller, manageable steps and allocate specific time slots for each.

- **Mindfulness and Stress-Reduction Techniques:**
- **Purpose:** Helps in managing emotional fluctuations and maintaining mental clarity.
- **Method:** Practice mindfulness meditation, deep breathing exercises, or yoga. These techniques can alleviate stress and improve focus.

- **Seek Professional Support:**

- **Purpose:** Provides guidance and strategies tailored to individual needs.
- **Method:** Engage with ADHD coaches, therapists, or support groups. Professional support can offer personalized strategies and emotional support.

- **Build a Support Network:**
- **Purpose:** Creates a safety net for times when additional help is needed.
- **Method:** Connect with friends, family members, or other parents who understand ADHD. Having a reliable support system can relieve some of the pressures of parenting.

- **Prioritize Tasks and Learn to Say No:**
- **Purpose:** Prevents overcommitment and reduces stress.
- **Method:** Identify the most critical tasks each day and focus on completing them first. Learn to decline additional responsibilities that may overwhelm your capacity.

Balancing ADHD Management with Parenting Responsibilities: A Case Study

Case Study: Lisa's Journey to Balanced Parenting
Lisa, a 32-year-old marketing professional and mother of two, was diagnosed with ADHD in her late twenties. Before her diagnosis, Lisa struggled with organization, time management,

and emotional regulation, often feeling overwhelmed by both her career and her parenting duties. Her undiagnosed ADHD led to missed deadlines at work, forgotten appointments, and strained relationships with her children.

Upon diagnosis, Lisa embarked on a journey to manage her ADHD symptoms more effectively while striving to be a present and organized mother. Here's how she achieved a balance:

Establishing a Structured Routine:

- Lisa implemented a daily schedule that included dedicated time blocks for work, household tasks, and family activities. This structure provided predictability for both her and her children, reducing chaos and improving efficiency.

Using Technology to Her Advantage:

- She started using a digital planner synced across all family members' devices. Reminders and alarms kept everyone on track, ensuring that tasks and appointments were not forgotten.

Delegating and Sharing Responsibilities:

- Lisa involved her partner and older child in household chores, creating a collaborative environment. This not only lightened her load but also fostered a sense of responsibility among her children.

Prioritizing Self-Care:

- Recognizing the importance of self-care, Lisa made time for regular exercise and mindfulness practices. These activities helped her manage stress and maintain focus throughout the day.

Seeking Professional Support:

- Lisa worked with an ADHD coach who helped her develop personalized strategies for managing her time and responsibilities. Additionally, she attended a support group for parents with ADHD, gaining insights and encouragement from others facing similar challenges.

Creating an Organized Home Environment:

- She decluttered her home, establishing designated areas for essential items. Simple organizational systems, such as labeled bins and drawers, made it easier to keep the household running smoothly.

Setting Realistic Goals:

- Lisa set achievable, incremental goals for both her personal and professional life. Celebrating small successes boosted her confidence and motivated her to continue improving.

Through these strategies, Lisa was able to transform her parenting approach and manage her ADHD symptoms more effectively. Her home became a more organized and peaceful environment, and her relationships with her children improved significantly. Lisa's story illustrates that with the right tools and support, it is possible to balance personal ADHD management with the demands of parenting.

Building a Supportive Family Environment

Creating a supportive family environment is crucial for parents with ADHD. It not only aids in the effective management of ADHD symptoms but also fosters healthy relationships and a positive atmosphere for children to thrive.

Educate Family Members About ADHD:

- **Purpose:** Promotes understanding and empathy, reducing the likelihood of misinterpretations and conflicts.
- **Method:** Share resources and information about ADHD with family members. Encourage open discussions about how ADHD affects daily life and family dynamics.

Establish Open Communication:

- **Purpose:** Ensures that everyone in the family feels heard and supported.
- **Method:** Create forums for family members to express their feelings, concerns, and needs. Regular family meetings can facilitate this open communication.

Model Healthy Behaviors:

- **Purpose:** Sets a positive example for children, teaching them effective coping strategies and organizational skills.
- **Method:** Demonstrate time management, organization, and stress-reduction techniques. Let children observe and

learn from these practices.

Encourage Independence in Children:

- **Purpose:** Empowers children to take responsibility for their tasks, reducing the burden on the parent.
- **Method:** Assign age-appropriate chores and responsibilities. Use visual aids like charts and checklists to guide them in completing tasks independently.

Foster a Positive and Supportive Atmosphere:

- **Purpose:** Creates a nurturing environment where children feel safe and supported.
- **Method:** Celebrate family achievements, practice gratitude, and maintain a positive outlook even during challenging times.

Tailoring Parenting Strategies to ADHD Strengths

While ADHD presents challenges, it also brings unique strengths that can enhance parenting:

Creativity and Spontaneity:

- **Benefit:** Can lead to innovative solutions and engaging activities for children.
- **Implementation:** Incorporate creative problem-solving methods and spontaneous fun into family routines to keep interactions lively and enjoyable.

Hyperfocus:

- **Benefit:** Allows for intense concentration on tasks of interest, which can be leveraged for meaningful activities with children.
- **Implementation:** Use periods of hyperfocus to engage deeply with children's projects, helping them with homework or creative endeavors.

High Energy Levels:

- **Benefit:** Can translate into active and dynamic family activities.
- **Implementation:** Organize physical activities, such as sports or outdoor adventures, that utilize and channel energy positively.

Empathy and Intuition:

- **Benefit:** Enhances emotional connections and understanding of children's needs.
- **Implementation:** Foster open emotional communication, providing a supportive space for children to express their feelings and experiences.

Overcoming Common Parenting Challenges with ADHD

Despite the strategies in place, parents with ADHD may still face specific challenges. Here are ways to address some common issues:

Forgetfulness and Missed Appointments:

- **Solution:** Implement a robust reminder system using digital calendars and alarms. Keep a visible family calendar to track important dates and events.

Inconsistent Discipline:

- **Solution:** Develop clear and consistent rules for children. Use visual aids and discussion to reinforce expectations, ensuring that disciplinary actions are predictable and fair.

Difficulty in Multitasking:

- **Solution:** Focus on one task at a time, breaking down larger tasks into manageable steps. Prioritize activities to ensure that essential tasks are completed without overwhelming yourself.

Emotional Volatility:

- **Solution:** Practice emotional regulation techniques such as deep breathing, mindfulness, or taking short breaks to cool down before addressing challenging situations with children.

Leveraging Professional and Community Resources

Parents with ADHD can significantly benefit from various professional and community resources designed to support their unique needs:

Therapists and Coaches Specializing in ADHD:

- **Benefit:** Provide personalized strategies and support for managing ADHD symptoms in the context of parenting.
- **Access:** Seek professionals with experience in ADHD and family dynamics, ensuring that guidance is tailored to specific challenges.

Parenting Workshops and Programs:

- **Benefit:** Offer practical tools and techniques for effective parenting, often incorporating ADHD-friendly approaches.
- **Access:** Enroll in local or online workshops that focus on ADHD and parenting, providing opportunities to learn and connect with others.

Support Groups:

- **Benefit:** Create a sense of community and shared experiences, reducing feelings of isolation.
- **Access:** Join ADHD support groups, either in-person or online, to share experiences, exchange advice, and build a supportive network.

Educational Resources:

- **Benefit:** Enhance understanding of ADHD and its impact on parenting, facilitating better management strategies.
- **Access:** Utilize books, articles, and reputable websites dedicated to ADHD and parenting. Regularly update knowledge with the latest research and best practices.

Community Services:

- **Benefit:** Provide additional support for both parents and children, such as childcare assistance, counseling services, and educational support.
- **Access:** Explore local community centers and non-profit organizations that offer services tailored to families dealing with ADHD.

Conclusion: Embracing the Journey with ADHD

Parenting with ADHD entails navigating a complex landscape of personal and familial responsibilities. However, with the right strategies, support systems, and self-awareness, it is entirely possible to balance personal needs with effective childcare. Embracing both the challenges and strengths that come with ADHD can lead to a fulfilling and harmonious family life.

Key Takeaways:

- **Structured Routines:** Implementing consistent and visually clear routines can reduce chaos and provide a sense of stability for the entire family.
- **Effective Use of Technology:** Leveraging digital tools and reminders can compensate for organizational challenges, ensuring that important tasks and appointments are not overlooked.
- **Delegation and Support:** Sharing responsibilities and seeking support from partners, family members, and professional resources can alleviate the pressures of parenting.
- **Prioritization and Self-Care:** Recognizing the importance

of self-care and prioritizing tasks helps maintain personal well-being and enhances parenting effectiveness.

· **Harnessing ADHD Strengths:** Utilizing the creative, energetic, and empathetic qualities associated with ADHD can enrich the parenting experience and foster stronger family bonds.

By acknowledging and addressing the unique intersection of ADHD and parenting, women can cultivate a nurturing environment that supports both their personal growth and their children's development. This balanced approach not only enhances the quality of life for the parent but also lays the foundation for a resilient and thriving family unit.

8

Health and Wellness: Creating an ADHD-Friendly Lifestyle

Living with Attention Deficit Hyperactivity Disorder (ADHD) presents unique challenges, particularly when it comes to maintaining physical health and overall wellness. For women with ADHD, managing symptoms often requires a multifaceted approach that includes not only medical treatments but also lifestyle adjustments. Chapter 8 delves into the intricate relationship between ADHD and physical health, exploring how nutrition, exercise, sleep, and other wellness practices can significantly influence symptom management and quality of life. Through personal anecdotes and detailed case studies, this chapter provides practical strategies for creating an ADHD-friendly lifestyle tailored to the needs of women.

Introduction: The Holistic Connection Between Health and ADHD

ADHD is commonly associated with difficulties in concentration, hyperactivity, and impulsivity. However, the disorder's impact extends far beyond mental focus, influencing various aspects of physical health and daily living. For women, hormonal fluctuations, societal roles, and unique psychological traits interplay with ADHD symptoms, necessitating a personalized approach to health and wellness.

A holistic lifestyle that addresses nutrition, physical activity, sleep, and stress management can serve as a powerful adjunct to traditional treatments like medication and therapy. By understanding and implementing ADHD-friendly health practices, women can enhance their ability to manage symptoms, boost their overall well-being, and lead fulfilling lives.

Nutrition and ADHD: Fueling the Brain and Body
The Role of Diet in ADHD Management
Nutrition plays a pivotal role in managing ADHD symptoms. The brain requires a steady supply of nutrients to function optimally, and dietary choices can influence neurotransmitter activity, energy levels, and cognitive performance. For women with ADHD, maintaining a balanced diet can help mitigate some of the challenges associated with the disorder.

Balanced Diet: The Foundation of Wellness
A balanced diet rich in whole foods—fruits, vegetables, lean proteins, whole grains, and healthy fats—provides essential vitamins and minerals that support brain health. Omega-3 fatty acids, found in fish, flaxseeds, and walnuts, are particularly beneficial for cognitive function and have been linked to reduced ADHD symptoms.

Key Nutrients for ADHD:

- **Protein:** Stabilizes blood sugar levels and enhances neurotransmitter production.

THE DEFINITIVE GUIDE TO ADHD FOR WOMEN

- **Complex Carbohydrates:** Provide a steady energy supply without causing spikes and crashes.
- **Vitamins and Minerals:** B-vitamins, iron, magnesium, and zinc are crucial for brain health and energy metabolism.

Foods to Embrace and Avoid

Certain foods can exacerbate ADHD symptoms, while others can help alleviate them. It's important for women with ADHD to be mindful of their dietary choices and how these choices affect their daily functioning.

Foods to Embrace:

- **Lean Proteins:** Chicken, turkey, tofu, and legumes.
- **Whole Grains:** Brown rice, quinoa, and oats.
- **Fruits and Vegetables:** Berries, leafy greens, and cruciferous vegetables.
- **Healthy Fats:** Avocados, nuts, and olive oil.

Foods to Avoid:

- **Sugary Snacks and Beverages:** Excess sugar can lead to energy crashes and increased hyperactivity.
- **Processed Foods:** High in additives and preservatives that may negatively impact behavior.
- **Caffeine and Artificial Stimulants:** Can interfere with sleep and exacerbate anxiety.

Case Study: Dietary Transformation Enhances Focus

Emily's Journey to Better Focus through Nutrition

Emily, a 35-year-old graphic designer, struggled with ADHD symptoms that affected her productivity and creativity. Despite trying various medications, she found limited improvement and experienced unwanted side effects. Determined to find alternative strategies, Emily consulted a nutritionist specialized in ADHD.

Together, they devised a meal plan emphasizing whole foods, high in protein and omega-3 fatty acids. Emily eliminated processed snacks and incorporated more fruits, vegetables, and lean proteins into her diet. Within a few weeks, she noticed significant improvements in her concentration and overall energy levels. The dietary changes not only reduced her ADHD symptoms but also enhanced her mood and motivation, empowering her to excel in her professional and personal life.

Exercise and ADHD: Harnessing Physical Activity for Mental Clarity

The Benefits of Regular Physical Activity

Exercise is a powerful tool in managing ADHD symptoms. Physical activity stimulates the release of endorphins, which can enhance mood, reduce stress, and improve focus. For women with ADHD, incorporating regular exercise into their routines can lead to better symptom control and overall well-being.

Benefits of Exercise for ADHD:

- **Improved Concentration:** Increased blood flow to the brain enhances cognitive functions.
- **Stress Reduction:** Physical activity helps mitigate anxiety and depression, which are commonly comorbid with ADHD.

- **Enhanced Mood:** Endorphins released during exercise contribute to a sense of well-being and happiness.

Types of Exercise That Help

Not all exercises are created equal when it comes to managing ADHD. Women with ADHD may find certain types of physical activity more beneficial in addressing their specific needs.

Recommended Exercises:

- **Aerobic Activities:** Running, cycling, and swimming increase heart rate and promote mental clarity.
- **Strength Training:** Lifting weights or using resistance bands can improve focus and discipline.
- **Mind-Body Practices:** Yoga and Pilates combine physical movement with mindfulness, aiding in stress reduction and concentration.

Anecdote: Integrating Exercise into a Busy Schedule

Sarah's Story: Finding Time for Fitness

Sarah, a single mother and marketing executive, struggled to find time for exercise amidst her demanding schedule. Her ADHD made it challenging to adhere to a consistent routine, often leading to feelings of overwhelm and fatigue. Determined to improve her health, Sarah decided to incorporate short, manageable workouts into her day.

She started with 15-minute morning yoga sessions, which helped her center her thoughts and prepare for the day ahead.

In the evenings, Sarah engaged in brisk walks with her children, combining physical activity with quality family time. These small adjustments not only improved her physical health but also enhanced her mental clarity and emotional resilience, allowing her to navigate her busy life more effectively.

Sleep and ADHD: Ensuring Restful Nights for Productive Days
The Importance of Quality Sleep
Sleep is crucial for cognitive function, emotional regulation, and overall health. Women with ADHD are more likely to experience sleep disturbances, which can exacerbate symptoms such as inattention, irritability, and impulsivity. Establishing healthy sleep habits is essential for managing ADHD effectively.

Common Sleep Challenges in ADHD
Women with ADHD may face several sleep-related issues, including:

- **Difficulty Falling Asleep:** Racing thoughts and restlessness can make it hard to wind down at night.
- **Poor Sleep Quality:** Frequent awakenings and light sleep can lead to feeling unrefreshed.
- **Irregular Sleep Patterns:** Inconsistent sleep schedules can disrupt the body's internal clock.

Strategies for Improving Sleep Hygiene
Implementing good sleep hygiene practices can significantly enhance sleep quality for women with ADHD. Here are some effective strategies:

- **Consistent Sleep Schedule:** Going to bed and waking up at the same time each day helps regulate the body's internal clock.
- **Relaxing Bedtime Routine:** Engaging in calming activities, such as reading or taking a warm bath, can prepare the mind and body for sleep.
- **Limiting Screen Time:** Reducing exposure to screens at least an hour before bedtime can prevent disruptions to melatonin production.
- **Creating a Sleep-Friendly Environment:** A cool, dark, and quiet bedroom promotes better sleep.

Case Study: Overcoming Insomnia through Routine and Relaxation

Linda's Battle with Sleep and Her Path to Restful Nights

Linda, a 29-year-old teacher, struggled with chronic insomnia that left her exhausted and unable to concentrate during the day. Her ADHD exacerbated her sleep issues, creating a vicious cycle of fatigue and inattention. Seeking help, Linda worked with a sleep specialist and a therapist to develop a comprehensive sleep plan.

They established a strict sleep schedule, ensuring she went to bed and woke up at the same time every day. Linda incorporated a calming bedtime routine, including meditation and gentle stretching, to signal her body that it was time to wind down. She also made changes to her sleep environment, using blackout curtains and white noise machines to create a restful atmosphere.

Within a few weeks, Linda experienced significant improvements in her sleep quality. She felt more rested, her concentration in the classroom improved, and her overall mood became more stable. By prioritizing sleep, Linda was able to break the cycle of exhaustion and better manage her ADHD symptoms.

Overall Wellness Practices: Building a Foundation for a Balanced Life

Stress Management Techniques

Chronic stress can worsen ADHD symptoms, making stress management a crucial component of an ADHD-friendly lifestyle. Women with ADHD can benefit from various stress-reduction techniques that promote relaxation and emotional resilience.

Effective Stress Management Practices:

- **Mindfulness Meditation:** Enhances present-moment awareness and reduces anxiety.
- **Deep Breathing Exercises:** Helps calm the nervous system and lower stress levels.
- **Progressive Muscle Relaxation:** Alleviates physical tension and promotes relaxation.

The Importance of Routine and Organization

Establishing a consistent daily routine can provide structure and predictability, which are beneficial for managing ADHD symptoms. Organizational strategies help reduce chaos and improve productivity, making it easier to stay on track with personal and professional responsibilities.

Organizational Tips:

- **Use Calendars and Planners:** Keep track of appointments, deadlines, and tasks.
- **Declutter Regularly:** Maintain a tidy living and working space to minimize distractions.
- **Set Priorities:** Focus on the most important tasks and break them into manageable steps.

Mind-Body Practices

Integrating mind-body practices into daily life can enhance mental clarity and emotional well-being. These practices bridge the gap between physical health and cognitive function, offering a holistic approach to ADHD management.

Recommended Mind-Body Practices:

- **Yoga:** Combines physical movement with breath control and mindfulness.
- **Tai Chi:** Promotes balance, flexibility, and mental focus.
- **Pilates:** Enhances core strength and body awareness.

Creating an ADHD-Friendly Lifestyle: Practical Tips and Strategies

Developing an ADHD-friendly lifestyle involves making intentional choices that support physical health and overall well-being. Here are some practical tips to help women with ADHD create a balanced and healthy life:

1. **Plan and Prepare Meals:** Dedicate time each week to plan

nutritious meals and prepare ingredients in advance. This reduces the likelihood of unhealthy eating habits driven by impulsivity or time constraints.

2. **Schedule Regular Exercise:** Incorporate physical activity into your daily routine, even if it's just a short walk or a quick workout session. Consistency is key to reaping the benefits of exercise.

3. **Prioritize Sleep:** Make sleep a non-negotiable part of your routine. Implement sleep hygiene practices and address any underlying sleep disorders with professional help if needed.

4. **Manage Stress Proactively:** Identify stress triggers and develop strategies to cope with them. Regularly engage in activities that promote relaxation and mental well-being.

5. **Maintain an Organized Environment:** Create a structured living and working space that minimizes distractions and fosters productivity. Use labeling, color-coding, and other organizational tools to keep things in order.

6. **Stay Hydrated and Limit Caffeine:** Proper hydration is essential for cognitive function. Limit caffeine intake, especially in the afternoon and evening, to prevent sleep disturbances.

7. **Seek Professional Guidance:** Work with healthcare providers, nutritionists, and fitness trainers who understand ADHD and can tailor their advice to your specific needs.

8. **Connect with Support Networks:** Engage with support groups, either in-person or online, to share experiences and gain insights from others managing ADHD.

Conclusion: Integrating Health and Wellness into Daily Life

Creating an ADHD-friendly lifestyle is a dynamic and on-going process that requires dedication and adaptability. By prioritizing nutrition, incorporating regular exercise, ensuring quality sleep, and adopting effective wellness practices, women with ADHD can significantly improve their ability to manage symptoms and enhance their overall quality of life.

The journey to wellness is unique for each individual, and what works for one person may not work for another. It is essential to experiment with different strategies, seek professional guidance, and remain patient and compassionate with oneself throughout the process. Embracing a holistic approach to health empowers women with ADHD to harness their strengths, overcome challenges, and thrive in all areas of life.

Anecdote: Integrating Exercise into a Busy Schedule

Sarah, a 32-year-old project manager and mother of two, found it incredibly challenging to incorporate exercise into her hectic daily routine. Her ADHD made it difficult to maintain a consistent schedule, and the demands of her job and family often left her drained by the end of the day. Determined to improve her energy levels and mental focus, Sarah decided to make small, manageable changes.

She began by dedicating just 10 minutes each morning to a series of stretching exercises and short yoga sessions. These brief workouts helped her wake up more fully and set a positive tone for the day. Additionally, Sarah incorporated physical activity into her family time by organizing weekend hikes and bike rides with her children. By integrating exercise into her existing commitments, Sarah was able to stay active without overwhelming her schedule. Over time, she noticed a significant improvement in her concentration, mood, and overall well-being, demonstrating that even small changes can have a profound impact.

Case Study: Dietary Changes Positively Impact ADHD Symptoms

Jessica's Dietary Overhaul Leads to Enhanced Cognitive Function

Jessica, a 28-year-old freelance writer, had long struggled with ADHD symptoms that hindered her productivity and creativity. She often felt mentally fatigued and found it hard to maintain focus on her projects. After years of trial and error with various medications, Jessica decided to explore the impact of her diet on her ADHD symptoms.

She consulted with a registered dietitian who specializes in ADHD and together, they crafted a meal plan emphasizing whole foods, lean proteins, and omega-3-rich foods. Jessica eliminated processed foods, refined sugars, and artificial additives from her diet. She also incorporated more leafy greens, nuts, seeds, and fatty fish into her meals.

Within a few weeks of making these dietary changes, Jessica experienced a noticeable improvement in her focus and mental clarity. Her energy levels became more stable throughout the day, and the foggy feeling that often accompanied her ADHD began to lift. By the end of three months, Jessica reported significant enhancements in her writing productivity and a greater sense of well-being. Her success illustrated the powerful role that nutrition can play in managing ADHD symptoms and emphasized the importance of a personalized approach to diet in ADHD treatment plans.

Final Thoughts

Chapter 8 of "The Definitive Guide to ADHD for Women" underscores the importance of a comprehensive approach to managing ADHD through health and wellness practices. By prioritizing nutrition, incorporating regular exercise, ensuring quality sleep, and adopting effective stress management techniques, women with ADHD can create a supportive environment that enhances their ability to thrive. Personal anecdotes and case studies provide relatable insights and practical examples, demonstrating that with intentional lifestyle changes, it is possible to improve ADHD symptoms and achieve a balanced, fulfilling life.

Embracing an ADHD-friendly lifestyle is not about perfection but about making consistent, small changes that collectively make a significant difference. As you integrate these strategies into your daily routine, remember to be patient with yourself and celebrate your progress. The journey to wellness is ongoing, and every step you take brings you closer to harnessing your strengths and living your best life.

9

Mindfulness and Alternative Therapies

In the multifaceted journey of managing ADHD, particularly for women who often navigate unique challenges, traditional treatments such as medication and cognitive-behavioral therapy (CBT) remain vital. However, an increasing body of evidence and personal testimonies highlights the significant benefits of integrating mindfulness practices and alternative therapies into ADHD management plans. This chapter delves into these complementary approaches, offering insights into their effectiveness, practical applications, and the transformative impact they can have on the lives of women with ADHD.

Understanding Mindfulness

Mindfulness is the practice of maintaining a nonjudgmental awareness of one's present moment experiences, encompassing thoughts, emotions, and physical sensations. Originating from ancient meditative traditions, mindfulness has been secularized and widely adopted in modern therapeutic settings due to its profound benefits on mental health.

For women with ADHD, mindfulness offers a respite from the

constant whirlwind of distractions and impulsivity. It cultivates an inner space where attention can be deliberately directed and sustained, counteracting the core symptoms of ADHD. Research has shown that mindfulness improves executive functions, such as working memory, cognitive flexibility, and inhibitory control—skills often compromised in individuals with ADHD.

Mindfulness Practices

1. Meditation

Meditation is a cornerstone of mindfulness, involving various techniques to focus attention and achieve mental clarity. For women with ADHD, meditation can be particularly challenging due to tendencies toward restlessness and difficulty sustaining attention. However, with practice, meditation can enhance focus and reduce the mental clutter that hinders productivity and emotional stability.

- **Guided Meditation:** This involves following a narrator or a recorded guide through the meditation process. It provides structure and focus, making it easier for beginners to engage.
- **Body Scan Meditation:** This practice directs attention to different parts of the body, promoting physical relaxation and heightened bodily awareness.
- **Breath Awareness Meditation:** Focusing solely on the breath helps anchor the mind, reducing the impact of intrusive thoughts and enhancing concentration.

2. Yoga

Yoga combines physical postures, breath control, and meditation, creating a holistic practice that benefits both the body and mind. For women with ADHD, yoga offers a structured yet flexible routine that can mitigate hyperactivity and impulsivity.

- **Hatha Yoga:** Emphasizes physical postures and breath control, fostering muscle strength and mental calmness.
- **Vinyasa Yoga:** Involves flowing movements synchronized with the breath, promoting fluidity and reducing mental rigidity.
- **Restorative Yoga:** Focuses on relaxation and stress relief, providing a sanctuary of calm amidst ADHD-related chaos.

3. Breathing Exercises

Controlled breathing techniques can significantly enhance focus and reduce anxiety, common challenges for women with ADHD.

- **Deep Breathing:** Inhaling deeply through the nose, holding for a few seconds, and exhaling slowly can calm the nervous system.
- **Box Breathing:** Involves inhaling, holding, exhaling, and holding again for equal counts, promoting balance and focus.
- **Alternate Nostril Breathing:** Balancing the breath between nostrils can enhance mental clarity and emotional stability.

4. Mindful Movement

Mindful movement practices, such as Tai Chi and Qigong, integrate slow, deliberate movements with breath awareness, fostering a deep connection between mind and body. These practices enhance coordination, reduce stress, and improve overall mental resilience.

Alternative Therapies

Beyond mindfulness, various alternative therapies have shown promise in alleviating ADHD symptoms and improving quality of life for women. These therapies often address underlying factors such as stress, hormonal imbalances, and neurological functioning.

1. Acupuncture

Acupuncture, a traditional Chinese medicine practice, involves inserting thin needles into specific points on the body to balance the flow of energy (Qi). For ADHD, acupuncture aims to enhance focus, reduce hyperactivity, and alleviate associated anxiety and depression.

- **Mechanism:** Acupuncture is believed to modulate neurotransmitter levels, improve blood flow to the brain, and regulate the nervous system.
- **Evidence:** Some studies indicate that acupuncture can reduce ADHD symptoms, though more rigorous research is needed to establish its efficacy definitively.

2. Neurofeedback

Neurofeedback, also known as EEG biofeedback, is a cutting-edge therapy that trains individuals to regulate their brainwave activity. By monitoring brainwaves in real-time, participants learn to modify their neural patterns to enhance attention and reduce impulsivity.

- **Process:** During a neurofeedback session, sensors are

placed on the scalp to detect brain activity. Visual or auditory feedback is provided to help the individual recognize and alter their brainwave patterns.

- **Benefits:** Neurofeedback has been shown to improve attention span, reduce hyperactivity, and enhance overall cognitive functioning. It offers a non-invasive alternative to medication, with lasting effects.

3. Occupational Therapy

Occupational therapy focuses on developing practical skills to manage daily tasks and improve organizational abilities. For women with ADHD, occupational therapists can design personalized strategies to enhance productivity and reduce overwhelm.

- **Techniques:** Time management training, organizational systems, sensory integration, and executive functioning support.
- **Outcomes:** Improved ability to manage household responsibilities, maintain work performance, and achieve personal goals.

4. Dietary Supplements

Certain dietary supplements are believed to support brain health and mitigate ADHD symptoms. Common supplements include omega-3 fatty acids, zinc, magnesium, and iron.

- **Omega-3 Fatty Acids:** Essential for brain function, omega-3s can improve attention and cognitive performance.
- **Zinc and Magnesium:** These minerals play roles in neurotransmitter regulation and can reduce hyperactivity and

impulsivity.

- **Iron:** Adequate iron levels are necessary for dopamine production, which is often dysregulated in ADHD.

5. Chiropractic Care

Chiropractic adjustments aim to correct spinal misalignments and enhance overall nervous system function. Some proponents suggest that chiropractic care can improve focus and reduce ADHD symptoms by optimizing neurological health.

- **Controversy:** While some individuals report benefits, scientific evidence supporting chiropractic care for ADHD is limited and mixed.

Combining Mindfulness and Alternative Therapies with Traditional Treatments

Integrating mindfulness and alternative therapies with conventional treatments can offer a more comprehensive approach to managing ADHD. This holistic strategy addresses not only the neurological aspects of ADHD but also the emotional, physical, and environmental factors that influence overall well-being.

- **Complementary Role:** Mindfulness practices can enhance the effectiveness of medication by improving adherence and reducing side effects. Alternative therapies like neurofeedback can work synergistically with CBT to provide deeper cognitive and behavioral changes.
- **Personalization:** Each individual's ADHD experience is unique, necessitating a tailored combination of treatments. Collaborating with healthcare providers ensures that mind-

fulness and alternative therapies are safely and effectively integrated into one's treatment plan.

Personal Accounts: Women Finding Relief Through Mindfulness

Anecdote 1: Sarah's Journey with Meditation

Sarah, a 34-year-old graphic designer, struggled with chronic restlessness and difficulty concentrating at work. Traditional treatments provided some relief, but she yearned for a sustainable way to manage her symptoms without relying solely on medication. Sarah turned to meditation, starting with guided sessions on a smartphone app. Initially, she found it challenging to sit still and quiet her mind. However, with consistent practice, Sarah noticed significant improvements in her focus and a reduction in anxiety. Meditating for just ten minutes each morning became a cornerstone of her daily routine, empowering her to approach her work with greater clarity and calm.

Anecdote 2: Jenna's Embrace of Yoga

Jenna, a single mother and freelance writer, faced the overwhelming demands of managing her household and career while contending with ADHD symptoms. Physical activity often left her feeling exhausted rather than invigorated, but she discovered yoga through a friend's recommendation. Jenna began attending beginner classes, initially struggling to keep up with the sequences. Over time, the combination of mindful movement and breath control helped her channel her energy more effectively. Yoga not only improved her physical stamina but also provided a mental sanctuary where she could decompress and regain focus, enhancing her productivity and emotional resilience.

Case Study: Neurofeedback in Reducing ADHD Symptoms

Case Study: Emily's Neurofeedback Experience

Emily, a 28-year-old marketing executive, experienced severe ADHD symptoms that impeded her career progression and strained her personal relationships. Conventional treatments, including stimulant medication and CBT, offered partial relief but left Emily seeking additional support. Her therapist recommended neurofeedback as a complementary therapy.

Initial Assessment: Emily underwent a comprehensive neurofeedback assessment, which revealed atypical brainwave patterns associated with ADHD—particularly in the areas governing attention and impulse control. A tailored neurofeedback protocol was developed, targeting these specific neural pathways.

Treatment Process: Over the course of 20 weekly sessions, Emily engaged in neurofeedback training, utilizing visual feedback on a computer screen to learn how to alter her brainwave activity. With each session, Emily became more adept at sustaining attention and resisting impulsive thoughts.

Outcomes: After completing the neurofeedback regimen, Emily reported a marked improvement in her ability to concentrate during meetings and presentations. Her impulsivity decreased, leading to more thoughtful decision-making both professionally and personally. Additionally, Emily experienced a reduction in anxiety levels, contributing to better overall mental health. Her neurofeedback experience underscored the potential of alternative therapies to enhance traditional ADHD treatments, providing a more holistic approach to symptom management.

Practical Tips for Incorporating Mindfulness and Alternative Therapies

Integrating mindfulness and alternative therapies into daily life requires intentionality and consistency. Here are practical strategies to help women with ADHD embrace these complementary approaches:

1. Start Small and Be Consistent

Begin with short, manageable sessions to avoid feeling overwhelmed. Even five minutes of mindfulness meditation or gentle yoga can create a foundation for more extended practices.

2. Choose Practices that Align with Your Interests and Lifestyle

Select mindfulness and alternative therapies that resonate with you personally. Whether it's dance-based movement, tai chi, or aromatherapy, finding joy in the practice increases the likelihood of sustained engagement.

3. Schedule Regular Practice Times

Incorporate mindfulness and alternative therapies into your daily routine by setting aside specific times for these activities. Consistency fosters habit formation and maximizes benefits.

4. Seek Professional Guidance

Working with trained practitioners—such as mindfulness instructors, yoga therapists, or neurofeedback specialists— can provide personalized support and ensure safe, effective practice.

5. Combine with Traditional Treatments

Use mindfulness and alternative therapies as complementary tools alongside traditional ADHD treatments. Communicate with your healthcare providers to create a cohesive and inte-grated treatment plan.

6. Monitor and Reflect on Progress

Keep a journal to track your experiences with mindfulness and alternative therapies. Reflecting on your progress can reinforce positive changes and identify areas for adjustment.

7. Be Patient and Persistent

Mindfulness and alternative therapies often require time to show their full benefits. Maintain patience and perseverance, recognizing that gradual improvements contribute to long-term well-being.

Conclusion

Mindfulness and alternative therapies offer invaluable tools for women with ADHD, complementing traditional treatments and fostering a holistic approach to symptom management. By embracing practices such as meditation, yoga, and neurofeed-back, women can cultivate greater focus, emotional resilience, and overall well-being. Personal accounts and case studies underscore the transformative potential of these approaches, highlighting their role in empowering women to navigate the complexities of ADHD with grace and strength.

As the understanding of ADHD in women continues to evolve, integrating mindfulness and alternative therapies becomes increasingly recognized as a vital component of comprehensive care. By exploring and adopting these complementary practices, women with ADHD can unlock new pathways to personal growth, enhanced functioning, and a more balanced, fulfilling life.

In this chapter, we have explored how mindfulness and alternative therapies can serve as powerful adjuncts to traditional ADHD treatments for women. By adopting these practices, women can harness their innate strengths, mitigate symptoms, and cultivate a deeper sense of self-awareness and control. The journey toward managing ADHD is uniquely personal, and embracing a diverse toolkit of strategies ensures that each woman can find the right balance to thrive.

10

Medical Treatments and Interventions

Navigating the medical landscape of Attention Deficit Hyper-activity Disorder (ADHD) can be a daunting journey, especially for women who often face unique challenges in diagnosis and treatment. Chapter 10 delves into the various medical treatments and interventions available for ADHD, providing a comprehensive overview of medication options, their benefits, potential side effects, and the critical importance of person-alized treatment plans. Through the exploration of personal stories and detailed case studies, this chapter aims to equip women with the knowledge needed to make informed decisions about their ADHD management.

Understanding ADHD Medications

Stimulant Medications
Stimulant medications are the most commonly prescribed treatments for ADHD and have been extensively studied for their efficacy. They work by increasing the levels of certain

neurotransmitters in the brain, particularly dopamine and norepinephrine, which are crucial for attention and focus.

Types of Stimulants:

1. **Methylphenidate-Based Medications:**

- **Ritalin®**
- **Concerta®**
- **Metadate®**

1. **Amphetamine-Based Medications:**

- **Adderall®**
- **Vyvanse®**
- **Dexedrine®**

Benefits:

- **Enhanced Focus and Attention:** Many women report significant improvements in concentration and the ability to sustain attention on tasks.
- **Improved Executive Function:** Stimulants can aid in organizing tasks, managing time, and prioritizing responsibilities.
- **Behavioral Regulation:** Reduced impulsivity and hyperactivity, contributing to better personal and professional relationships.

Potential Side Effects:

- **Physical:** Insomnia, decreased appetite, increased heart rate, and headaches.
- **Psychological:** Anxiety, mood swings, and, in rare cases, exacerbation of symptoms like agitation.

Non-Stimulant Medications

For those who do not respond well to stimulants or experience adverse side effects, non-stimulant medications offer an alternative.

Types of Non-Stimulants:

1. **Atomoxetine (Strattera®):** A selective norepinephrine reuptake inhibitor.
2. **Guanfacine (Intuniv®):** Originally developed for high blood pressure, it also treats ADHD symptoms.
3. **Clonidine (Kapvay®):** Another antihypertensive that is used off-label for ADHD.

Benefits:

- **Longer-Lasting Effects:** Some non-stimulants offer symptom control throughout the day without the need for multiple doses.
- **Lower Abuse Potential:** Non-stimulants are less likely to be misused or lead to dependency.
- **Fewer Sleep Disturbances:** Generally cause fewer issues with insomnia compared to stimulants.

Potential Side Effects:

- **Fatigue:** Some users may feel drowsy or tired.
- **Gastrointestinal Issues:** Nausea, vomiting, or stomach pain.
- **Mood Changes:** Potential for irritability or mood swings.

Other Medical Interventions

Beyond medications, several other medical interventions can assist in managing ADHD symptoms.

1. **Behavioral Therapy:** Often used in conjunction with medication, behavioral therapy helps in developing coping strategies and improving organizational skills.
2. **Cognitive Behavioral Therapy (CBT):** Focuses on changing negative thought patterns and behaviors associated with ADHD.
3. **Neurofeedback:** A type of biofeedback that aims to train the brain to improve attention and reduce hyperactivity.

Personalized Treatment Plans

One of the most critical aspects of managing ADHD is recognizing that treatment is not one-size-fits-all. Personalized treatment plans consider the individual's unique symptoms, lifestyle, health conditions, and personal preferences.

Factors Influencing Treatment Choices

1. **Comorbid Conditions:** Many women with ADHD also

experience anxiety, depression, or other mental health conditions, which can influence medication choices.

2. **Lifestyle and Daily Routines:** Those with demanding schedules may benefit from long-acting medications to provide all-day symptom control.

3. **Side Effect Profiles:** Personal tolerance to certain side effects plays a significant role in selecting the appropriate medication.

4. **Genetic Factors:** Some individuals may metabolize medications differently, necessitating adjustments in dosage or type.

The Importance of Collaboration

Effective ADHD management requires a collaborative approach involving healthcare providers, patients, and often family members. Regular consultations and open communication ensure that the treatment plan evolves with the individual's changing needs.

Personal Stories: Navigating Medication Choices

Sarah's Journey with ADHD Medications

Sarah, a 35-year-old graphic designer, was diagnosed with ADHD in her early thirties after years of struggling with disorganization and chronic procrastination. Initially, Sarah was skeptical about medication, fearing the stigma and potential side effects.

Initial Trials: Sarah began with a low dose of **Adderall®**, an amphetamine-based stimulant. While she experienced improved focus and productivity, she also faced appetite suppression and mild anxiety. After discussing these side effects with her psychiatrist, Sarah transitioned to **Vyvanse®**, which provided a smoother onset and longer duration of effect with fewer anxiety symptoms.

Adjustments and Outcomes: Over time, Sarah worked with her healthcare provider to fine-tune her dosage. She also integrated **CBT** to address underlying anxiety. This combination allowed her to maintain productivity while managing side effects effectively. Sarah's story highlights the importance of patience and communication in finding the right medication regimen.

Emily's Switch from Stimulants to Non-Stimulants

Emily, a 28-year-old teacher, initially found relief with **Ritalin®**, a methylphenidate-based stimulant. However, she began experiencing significant insomnia and irritability, which impacted her teaching performance and personal life.

Transition to Non-Stimulants: After consulting with her healthcare provider, Emily started **Strattera® (atomoxetine)**. While the onset was slower compared to stimulants, Emily appreciated the steady symptom control without the disruptive side effects. Additionally, she noticed an improvement in her anxiety levels, which were previously exacerbated by stimulant use.

Balancing Treatment: Emily continues to work with her psychiatrist to monitor her response to Strattera, demonstrating that switching medications can sometimes provide a better balance between efficacy and quality of life.

Case Study: Comparing Treatment Approaches

Overview

This case study examines two women, Laura and Megan, both diagnosed with ADHD in their mid-twenties. Despite similar symptom profiles, their treatment approaches and outcomes differed significantly based on their chosen medical interventions.

Laura's Approach: Stimulant-Focused Treatment

Background: Laura is a 26-year-old marketing executive diagnosed with ADHD. Her primary symptoms include distractibility, impulsivity, and difficulty managing time.

Treatment Plan: Laura opted for a stimulant-based treatment, starting with **Concerta® (methylphenidate)**. The extended-release formulation allowed for once-daily dosing, aligning well with her busy work schedule.

Outcomes:

- **Benefits:** Laura experienced a marked improvement in focus and task completion. Her productivity at work increased, and she found it easier to manage deadlines.
- **Side Effects:** She noted a decrease in appetite and occasional headaches, which she managed by adjusting meal times and staying hydrated.

Adjustments: After six months, Laura worked with her doctor to adjust the dosage to optimize benefits while minimizing side effects. The collaborative approach ensured that her treatment remained effective and tolerable.

Megan's Approach: Integrative and Non-Stimulant Treatment

Background: Megan is a 27-year-old freelance writer who was diagnosed with ADHD after struggling with chronic disorganization and procrastination. She also has a history of anxiety.

Treatment Plan: Given her anxiety and sensitivity to stimulants, Megan chose a non-stimulant approach. She began with **Intuniv® (guanfacine)**, a non-stimulant medication, and incorporated **CBT** for both ADHD and anxiety management.

Outcomes:

- **Benefits:** Megan experienced a gradual improvement in her ability to focus and organize her tasks without the jitteriness associated with stimulants. Her anxiety levels also decreased with CBT.
- **Side Effects:** She reported mild drowsiness, especially during the initial weeks, which subsided as her body adjusted to the medication.

Adjustments: Megan and her healthcare provider monitored her progress closely, making dosage adjustments as needed. She also integrated mindfulness practices to further support her mental health.

Comparative Analysis

Both Laura and Megan achieved significant improvements in managing their ADHD symptoms. However, their experiences underscore the importance of individualized treatment plans:

- **Efficacy:** Both treatment approaches were effective, but

Laura benefited more from the immediate and robust symptom control provided by stimulants, while Megan found the non-stimulant approach more compatible with her anxiety.

- **Side Effect Management:** Laura managed her side effects through dosage adjustments, whereas Megan's side effects were minimal and self-limiting.
- **Complementary Therapies:** Megan's integration of CBT and mindfulness complemented her medication regimen, highlighting the value of combining medical and psychological interventions.

Navigating the Prescription Process

Securing the right medication involves a series of steps that require diligence, open communication, and patience.

Initial Consultation

The journey typically begins with a consultation with a health-care provider, often a psychiatrist or primary care physician, who specializes in ADHD. This consultation involves:

- **Comprehensive Evaluation:** Assessing ADHD symptoms, medical history, and any comorbid conditions.
- **Medication History:** Reviewing any past experiences with ADHD medications.
- **Personal Goals:** Understanding the patient's expectations and lifestyle to tailor the treatment plan accordingly.

Trial and Error

Finding the optimal medication often involves a period of trial and error. This phase may include:

- **Starting Low:** Initiating treatment with a low dose to monitor efficacy and side effects.
- **Gradual Increases:** Slowly adjusting the dosage based on the patient's response.
- **Monitoring:** Regular follow-ups to assess progress and make necessary modifications.

Ongoing Management

ADHD management is an ongoing process that may require:

- **Periodic Assessments:** Regular check-ins to evaluate the effectiveness of the treatment plan.
- **Adjustments:** Modifying dosages or switching medications based on changing needs or life circumstances.
- **Support Systems:** Incorporating therapy, coaching, and support groups to complement medical treatments.

Potential Side Effects and Mitigation Strategies

Understanding and managing side effects is crucial for maintaining adherence to the treatment plan and ensuring overall well-being.

Common Side Effects of Stimulants

Appetite Suppression:

· **Mitigation:** Encourage regular, balanced meals and con-sider scheduling meals before medication doses.

Insomnia:

· **Mitigation:** Take medications earlier in the day and estab-lish a consistent bedtime routine.

Increased Heart Rate:

· **Mitigation:** Regular cardiovascular exercise can help man-age heart rate, and consultation with a healthcare provider is essential if symptoms persist.

Mood Swings:

· **Mitigation:** Incorporate stress-reduction techniques such as mindfulness or yoga, and discuss persistent mood changes with a healthcare provider.

Common Side Effects of Non-Stimulants

Drowsiness:

· **Mitigation:** Taking the medication in the evening or ad-justing the dosage can help manage daytime drowsiness.

Gastrointestinal Issues:

- **Mitigation:** Taking medication with food and staying hydrated can alleviate stomach discomfort.

Dizziness:

- **Mitigation:** Rise slowly from sitting or lying positions to minimize dizziness and discuss persistent issues with a healthcare provider.

The Role of Healthcare Providers

Healthcare providers play a pivotal role in the successful management of ADHD. Their responsibilities include:

1. **Diagnosis and Evaluation:** Accurately diagnosing ADHD and identifying any comorbid conditions.
2. **Medication Management:** Prescribing appropriate medications, adjusting dosages, and monitoring for side effects.
3. **Collaborative Planning:** Working with patients to develop personalized treatment plans that align with their goals and lifestyles.
4. **Education and Support:** Providing information about ADHD, treatment options, and coping strategies, and referring patients to additional resources as needed.

Alternative and Complementary Treatments

While medications are a cornerstone of ADHD management, many women find that integrating alternative and complementary treatments enhances their overall strategy.

Neurofeedback

Neurofeedback, also known as EEG biofeedback, involves training individuals to modify their brain wave patterns. It is a non-invasive technique that can improve attention, reduce impulsivity, and enhance emotional regulation.

Benefits:

- **Non-Invasive:** No medications or external substances are required.
- **Long-Term Improvements:** Potential for lasting changes in brain function.

Considerations:

- **Accessibility:** Neurofeedback requires specialized equipment and trained practitioners.
- **Time Commitment:** Typically involves multiple sessions over an extended period.

Dietary Supplements

Certain dietary supplements, such as omega-3 fatty acids, have been explored for their potential benefits in managing ADHD symptoms.

Benefits:

- **Supportive Nutrients:** Omega-3s play a role in brain health and cognitive function.
- **Fewer Side Effects:** Generally well-tolerated with minimal adverse effects.

Considerations:

- **Efficacy:** While some studies show benefits, dietary supplements should not replace prescribed medications.
- **Consultation:** Always consult a healthcare provider before adding supplements to ensure they do not interact with other medications.

Mindfulness and Meditation

Mindfulness practices and meditation can enhance self-awareness, reduce stress, and improve focus, complementing medical treatments for ADHD.

Benefits:

- **Stress Reduction:** Lowering stress levels can mitigate ADHD-related anxiety and improve overall well-being.
- **Enhanced Focus:** Regular practice can train the brain to maintain attention and resist distractions.

Considerations:

- **Consistency:** Benefits are achieved through regular and sustained practice.
- **Integration:** Should be used as a complementary strategy alongside other treatments.

Barriers to Accessing Medical Treatments

Despite the availability of effective treatments, several barriers can impede access to appropriate medical interventions for ADHD.

Stigma and Misconceptions

Societal stigma surrounding ADHD and mental health can discourage women from seeking diagnosis and treatment. Misconceptions about ADHD being a condition that only affects children or not being "real" can lead to underdiagnosis and undertreatment.

Overcoming Stigma:

- **Education:** Raising awareness about ADHD in women can help dismantle harmful stereotypes.
- **Support Systems:** Encouraging open discussions within families and communities can foster a more supportive environment.

Financial Constraints

The cost of medications and ongoing healthcare can be prohibitive, especially for those without adequate insurance coverage.

Addressing Financial Barriers:

- **Insurance Navigation:** Working with healthcare providers to find covered medications.
- **Assistance Programs:** Exploring patient assistance programs and generic medication options to reduce costs.

Lack of Specialized Care

Access to healthcare providers who specialize in ADHD, particularly for women, can be limited, especially in underserved areas.

Enhancing Access:

- **Telehealth Services:** Utilizing telemedicine to connect with ADHD specialists remotely.
- **Advocacy:** Supporting initiatives that increase the availability of specialized ADHD care.

The Future of ADHD Treatment for Women

Advancements in medical research continue to enhance the understanding and treatment of ADHD, particularly for women who have historically been underrepresented in studies.

Personalized Medicine

The future of ADHD treatment lies in personalized medicine, which tailors interventions based on individual genetic makeup, lifestyle, and specific symptom profiles. This approach promises more effective and targeted treatments with reduced side effects.

Ongoing Research

Continued research into the neurobiological underpinnings of ADHD in women will lead to more refined and efficacious treatment options. Emerging therapies, such as gene therapy and advanced neurostimulation techniques, hold potential for future breakthroughs.

Increased Representation

Greater representation of women in ADHD research ensures that treatment protocols address the distinct needs of female patients. This shift will lead to more accurate diagnoses and tailored interventions that improve quality of life.

Conclusion

Chapter 10 has provided a thorough exploration of the medical treatments and interventions available for women with ADHD. From stimulant and non-stimulant medications to complementary therapies like neurofeedback and mindfulness, the spectrum of treatment options offers hope and practical solutions for managing ADHD symptoms. The personal stories of Sarah and Emily, along with the comparative case study of Laura and Megan, underscore the importance of individualized treatment plans and the need for ongoing collaboration with healthcare providers.

As women navigate their ADHD journeys, understanding the benefits and potential side effects of various treatments is crucial. By staying informed and proactive in seeking personalized care, women can effectively manage their symptoms, enhance their well-being, and thrive in both personal and professional arenas. The landscape of ADHD treatment is continually evolving, promising even greater support and innovation for women in the years to come.

Disclaimer: The information provided in this chapter is intended for educational purposes only and should not be construed as medical advice. Always consult with a qualified healthcare professional before starting or adjusting any treatment plan for ADHD.

11

Building a Support Network: Community and Resources

Introduction: The Power of Connection

Living with ADHD can often feel like navigating a labyrinth alone. The myriad challenges—from maintaining focus and managing time to handling emotional fluctuations—can be overwhelming. However, one of the most empowering strategies for managing ADHD is building a robust support network. For women with ADHD, who may face unique societal expectations and stereotypes, having a community that understands and supports them can make a significant difference in their personal and professional lives.

A strong support network provides emotional backing, practical advice, and a sense of belonging. It can help mitigate feelings of isolation, offer strategies for coping with daily challenges, and empower women to harness their strengths. This chapter delves into the various forms of support networks available, explores the benefits of each, and provides actionable tips on how to find and effectively utilize these resources.

The Importance of a Support Network

Before exploring the types of support networks, it's essential to understand why they are vital for women with ADHD:

1. **Emotional Support:** Dealing with ADHD-related challenges can lead to feelings of frustration, anxiety, and low self-esteem. A supportive community offers a safe space to express these emotions without judgment.

2. **Practical Strategies:** Sharing experiences within a community can lead to the exchange of effective coping mechanisms and organizational tips that have worked for others.

3. **Accountability:** Regular interactions with a support group or mentor can help maintain motivation and adherence to personal goals or treatment plans.

4. **Education and Awareness:** Being part of a network can enhance understanding of ADHD, dispel myths, and keep individuals informed about the latest research and resources.

5. **Advocacy and Empowerment:** A network can empower women to advocate for themselves in various settings, whether it's at work, in relationships, or within their communities.

Types of Support Networks

Support networks come in various forms, each offering unique benefits. Understanding the different types can help women with ADHD choose the ones that best fit their needs.

1. In-Person Support Groups

Description: Local groups where individuals meet regularly to share experiences, discuss challenges, and provide mutual support.

Benefits:

- **Face-to-Face Interaction:** Builds deeper connections and fosters a sense of community.
- **Structured Environment:** Often facilitated by a professional, ensuring productive discussions.
- **Consistent Meetings:** Provides routine and regular check-ins.

Finding In-Person Support Groups:

- **Local Mental Health Centers:** Many offer support groups for ADHD.
- **Community Centers and Libraries:** Frequently host meetings or have bulletin boards with information.
- **Non-Profit Organizations:** Organizations like CHADD (Children and Adults with Attention-Deficit/Hyperactivity Disorder) often have local chapters.

2. Online Communities

Description: Virtual platforms where individuals can connect, share, and support each other regardless of geographical location.

Benefits:

- **Accessibility:** Easy to join from anywhere, making it ideal

for those with mobility issues or busy schedules.
- **Anonymity:** Allows for more open sharing without the fear of being recognized.
- **Diverse Perspectives:** Connects women from different backgrounds and experiences.

Popular Online Platforms:

- **Social Media Groups:** Facebook, Reddit, and LinkedIn host numerous ADHD-focused groups.
- **Dedicated Forums:** Websites like ADHDSupport and ADDitude have active communities.
- **Online Support Apps:** Apps like MeetUp and Mighty Networks facilitate virtual gatherings.

3. Mentors and Coaches
Description: One-on-one relationships with experienced individuals who provide guidance, accountability, and personalized strategies.
Benefits:

- **Personalized Support:** Tailored advice and strategies based on individual needs.
- **Accountability:** Regular check-ins help maintain focus on goals.
- **Skill Development:** Coaches can teach specific skills for managing ADHD symptoms.

Finding Mentors and Coaches:

- **Professional Organizations:** CHADD and ADDA (Attention Deficit Disorder Association) offer directories.
- **Referrals from Healthcare Providers:** Therapists and psychiatrists often know reputable coaches.
- **Online Platforms:** Websites like LinkedIn and specialized coaching directories.

4. Professional Help

Description: Support from healthcare professionals, including therapists, psychologists, and psychiatrists, who specialize in ADHD.

Benefits:

- **Expert Guidance:** Access to evidence-based treatments and therapies.
- **Medical Management:** Professionals can prescribe and manage medications.
- **Comprehensive Care:** Addressing co-occurring conditions like anxiety or depression.

Accessing Professional Help:

- **Healthcare Providers:** Primary care doctors can provide referrals.
- **Specialized Clinics:** ADHD-focused clinics offer comprehensive services.
- **Telehealth Services:** Online therapy and consultations have become increasingly available.

Benefits of Each Support Network

Each type of support network offers distinct advantages, and the best approach often involves a combination of multiple resources.

- **In-Person Support Groups** offer the strength of community and shared experiences, fostering a sense of belonging and reducing isolation.
- **Online Communities** provide flexibility and reach, allowing connection with a broader range of individuals and resources.
- **Mentors and Coaches** deliver tailored guidance and accountability, essential for personal development and achieving specific goals.
- **Professional Help** ensures access to clinical expertise and medical interventions necessary for comprehensive management of ADHD.

By integrating these support networks, women with ADHD can create a multifaceted support system that addresses emotional, practical, and medical needs.

Finding and Choosing the Right Support Network

Navigating the vast array of available support networks can be daunting. Here are strategies to identify and select the most suitable resources:

1. Identify Your Needs

Start by assessing what you seek from a support network:

- **Emotional Support:** Look for groups focused on sharing and understanding personal experiences.
- **Practical Strategies:** Seek communities or coaches that emphasize skill-building and organizational techniques.
- **Professional Guidance:** Identify mental health professionals with expertise in ADHD.

2. Research Available Options

- **Local Resources:** Utilize online search engines, community bulletin boards, and local mental health centers to find in-person groups.
- **Online Platforms:** Explore forums, social media groups, and dedicated websites to find active online communities.
- **Professional Directories:** Use resources provided by organizations like CHADD or ADDA to find reputable coaches and therapists.

3. Evaluate the Community

- **Group Dynamics:** Attend a few meetings or participate in online discussions to gauge the group's compatibility with your personality and needs.
- **Facilitation Quality:** Ensure that support groups are well-facilitated, maintaining respectful and constructive dialogue.
- **Diversity and Inclusivity:** Choose communities that recognize and respect diverse backgrounds and experiences.

4. Seek Recommendations

- **Personal Referrals:** Ask friends, family, or healthcare providers for recommendations based on their experiences.
- **Online Reviews:** Read testimonials and reviews to understand others' experiences with specific groups or professionals.

5. Start Small and Adjust

- **Trial Participation:** Join a group or attend a coaching session to see if it meets your expectations.
- **Flexibility:** Be open to changing or trying different support networks if your initial choice doesn't resonate.

Utilizing Support Networks Effectively

Joining a support network is just the first step; maximizing its benefits requires active and intentional participation. Here are strategies to make the most of your support communities:

1. Be Open and Honest

- **Share Your Experiences:** Authentic sharing fosters deeper connections and mutual understanding.
- **Express Needs and Boundaries:** Clearly communicate what you seek and what you're comfortable sharing.

2. Engage Actively

- **Participate Regularly:** Consistent involvement helps build trust and rapport within the community.
- **Contribute:** Offer support, share resources, and provide feedback to others in the group.

3. Set Personal Goals

- **Identify Objectives:** Determine what you aim to achieve through the support network, such as improving organizational skills or building self-esteem.
- **Use Accountability:** Leverage the community to stay committed to your goals and track progress.

4. Utilize Available Resources

- **Educational Materials:** Take advantage of workshops, webinars, and literature provided by the group.
- **Networking Opportunities:** Connect with individuals who can offer additional support or resources outside the group.

5. Maintain Boundaries

- **Manage Expectations:** Understand that while support networks are beneficial, they are not substitutes for professional medical advice.
- **Self-Care:** Balance participation with personal well-being

to avoid burnout.

Anecdote: The Transformative Impact of Joining an ADHD Support Group

Emma's Journey to Connection and Clarity

Emma, a 35-year-old graphic designer, had been grappling with undiagnosed ADHD for years. Her struggles with time management, organization, and maintaining focus had taken a toll on her career and personal life. Despite her creative talents, Emma often felt overwhelmed and inadequate, attributing her difficulties to personal failings rather than understanding her ADHD.

Feeling isolated and desperate for change, Emma decided to join a local ADHD support group recommended by a colleague. Reluctantly, she attended her first meeting, unsure of what to expect. To her surprise, she found a circle of women who shared similar struggles and triumphs. As the sessions progressed, Emma felt a sense of belonging and validation she hadn't experienced before.

One particular meeting where members discussed balancing work and personal life resonated deeply with Emma. She learned practical strategies for prioritizing tasks and setting realistic goals. Moreover, hearing others share their stories of late diagnosis and the relief that came with understanding their ADHD provided Emma with newfound hope.

Inspired by the group's collective resilience, Emma began implementing the techniques she learned. Her productivity improved, and she developed healthier coping mechanisms for stress. The emotional support from the group also bolstered her self-esteem, empowering her to advocate for herself at work and in her relationships.

Emma's experience underscores the profound impact that a supportive community can have on women with ADHD. Through connection, shared wisdom, and mutual encouragement, support groups can transform lives, fostering both personal and professional growth.

Case Study: Leveraging Online Resources for ADHD Management

Samantha's Digital Journey to Empowerment

Samantha, a 28-year-old software engineer, was diagnosed with ADHD in her early twenties after years of struggling with disorganization and inattentiveness. While she received medical treatment, she felt the need for additional support to manage her symptoms effectively. With a demanding job and a busy social life, Samantha sought a flexible support system that could fit into her hectic schedule, leading her to explore online resources.

Exploring Online Communities

Samantha discovered several online ADHD communities, including a popular Facebook group and a dedicated forum on ADHDSupport.com. She appreciated the ability to engage with others at her own pace, posting questions and sharing experiences without the constraints of physical meetings.

Engaging with Online Coaching

In addition to community forums, Samantha enrolled in an

online ADHD coaching program. The virtual sessions provided personalized strategies for time management, goal setting, and maintaining focus. The coach also connected Samantha with other resources, such as productivity apps and mindfulness exercises tailored to ADHD.

Utilizing Educational Resources

Samantha took advantage of webinars and online workshops offered by ADHD organizations. These sessions covered topics like executive function skills, emotional regulation, and career advancement strategies, equipping her with a deeper understanding of her condition and practical tools to navigate challenges.

Building a Digital Support Network

Through her online interactions, Samantha connected with women worldwide who shared similar professional and personal interests. These connections extended beyond the forums, leading to virtual study groups, accountability partnerships, and even collaborative projects that leveraged their collective strengths.

Outcomes and Benefits

By leveraging online resources, Samantha experienced significant improvements in her ADHD management:

- **Enhanced Organization:** Implemented digital planners and task management tools recommended by the community.
- **Increased Productivity:** Adopted time-blocking techniques discussed in coaching sessions, leading to more efficient workdays.
- **Emotional Resilience:** Participated in virtual support meetings that provided emotional backing during stressful

periods.

· **Professional Growth:** Leveraged networking opportunities to advance her career, utilizing the collective knowledge of her online connections.

Samantha's case illustrates how online resources can offer comprehensive support for women with ADHD, providing flexibility, accessibility, and a wealth of information that empowers individuals to take control of their lives.

Building and Maintaining Your Support Network

Creating a support network is an ongoing process that requires intentional effort and commitment. Here are steps to build and sustain a robust support system:

1. Start Small

Begin by reaching out to one or two support groups or online communities to avoid feeling overwhelmed. Gradually expand your network as you become more comfortable.

2. Be Consistent

Regular participation is key to building trust and deepening connections. Schedule time each week to engage with your support networks.

3. Stay Open to New Connections

Be willing to explore different types of support networks, such as combining in-person groups with online communities or seeking both peer support and professional coaching.

4. Give Back

Contribute to your support networks by sharing your experiences and offering support to others. This reciprocal relationship enhances the strength and resilience of the community.

5. Evaluate and Adjust

Periodically assess the effectiveness of your support networks. If a particular group or resource no longer meets your needs, don't hesitate to seek alternatives.

Tips for Maximizing the Benefits of Your Support Network

To fully harness the advantages of your support network, consider the following tips:

1. Communicate Your Needs Clearly

Be upfront about what you hope to gain from the support network. Whether it's emotional support, practical advice, or accountability, clear communication ensures that your needs are met.

2. Set Boundaries

Maintain healthy boundaries to protect your well-being. Limit the time spent on support networks to prevent burnout and ensure that interactions remain positive and constructive.

3. Utilize Multiple Resources

Don't rely solely on one type of support network. Combining various resources—such as in-person groups, online communities, and professional help—provides a more comprehensive support system.

4. Stay Engaged and Active

Active participation enhances the benefits of support networks. Attend meetings regularly, engage in discussions, and take initiative in group activities.

5. Seek Professional Guidance When Needed

While support networks are invaluable, they complement rather than replace professional medical advice. Continue to consult with healthcare providers for comprehensive ADHD management.

Overcoming Common Challenges in Building a Support Network

While building a support network is beneficial, it can come with its own set of challenges. Here are strategies to overcome common obstacles:

1. Time Constraints

Challenge: Busy schedules can make consistent participation difficult.

Solution:

- **Prioritize:** Schedule dedicated time for support activities as part of your routine.
- **Choose Flexible Options:** Opt for online communities or support groups with flexible meeting times.
- **Set Realistic Goals:** Commit to manageable levels of participation to avoid feeling overwhelmed.

2. Finding the Right Fit

Challenge: Not every support group or community will align with your needs or personality.

Solution:

- **Explore Multiple Options:** Attend different groups or engage with various online communities to find a compatible fit.
- **Be Patient:** Building meaningful connections takes time; give yourself grace during the search process.
- **Seek Recommendations:** Ask trusted individuals or professionals for suggestions based on your specific needs.

3. Overcoming Stigma and Shame

Challenge: Societal stigma around ADHD can lead to feelings of shame, making it hard to seek support.

Solution:

- **Educate Yourself:** Understanding ADHD can empower you to overcome internalized stigma.
- **Connect with Empathetic Individuals:** Seek out groups that foster a non-judgmental and supportive environment.
- **Practice Self-Compassion:** Remind yourself that seeking support is a strength, not a weakness.

4. Maintaining Consistency

Challenge: Life changes, such as job transitions or family responsibilities, can disrupt participation.

Solution:

- **Adapt Your Support System:** Explore different formats, such as virtual meetings, to maintain engagement during life changes.
- **Communicate Your Needs:** Inform your support network about your situation to receive understanding and flexibility.
- **Re-establish Routine:** Gradually reintegrate support activities as your schedule stabilizes.

The Role of Technology in Enhancing Support Networks

In today's digital age, technology plays a pivotal role in expanding and enhancing support networks for women with ADHD. Here are ways technology can be leveraged:

1. Virtual Meetings and Webinars

Platforms like Zoom, Microsoft Teams, and Google Meet facilitate virtual support group meetings, making it easier to connect despite geographical barriers.

2. Mobile Apps

Apps designed for ADHD management, such as Todoist for task management, Headspace for mindfulness, or Habitica for building routines, can complement support network strategies.

3. Social Media

Social media platforms allow for real-time interactions, resource sharing, and community building. They also provide a space for advocacy and raising awareness about ADHD.

4. Online Learning Platforms

Websites like Coursera, Udemy, and Khan Academy offer courses on ADHD management, organizational skills, and personal development, providing valuable educational resources.

Expanding Your Support Beyond ADHD

While ADHD-specific support networks are invaluable, expanding your support system to include other aspects of your life can provide a more holistic approach to well-being.

1. Professional Networks

Connecting with colleagues and industry professionals can offer career guidance and support tailored to your professional aspirations.

2. Personal Interest Groups

Joining groups related to hobbies or interests, such as book clubs, sports teams, or art classes, can provide a balanced and fulfilling support network outside of ADHD.

3. Family and Friends

Engaging with family and friends who understand your ADHD and support your journey is crucial. Educate them about your condition to foster understanding and empathy.

Conclusion: Embracing Community and Support

Building a support network is a transformative step for

women with ADHD. It offers a sanctuary of understanding, a hub of practical strategies, and a platform for personal growth. Whether through in-person support groups, online communities, mentors, or professional help, each component of a support network contributes to a comprehensive and empowering approach to managing ADHD.

By actively seeking out and engaging with these resources, women with ADHD can overcome feelings of isolation, develop effective management strategies, and harness their unique strengths. The journey towards building a robust support network is gradual and requires patience, but the rewards— a sense of belonging, enhanced well-being, and greater self-empowerment—are invaluable.

As you embark on building your support network, remember that you are not alone. There are countless women and allies ready to join you on this journey, offering support, understanding, and shared wisdom. Embrace the power of community, and let it guide you towards a thriving and fulfilling life with ADHD.

Key Takeaways

- **Identify and Understand Needs:** Recognize what you seek from a support network to choose the most appropriate resources.
- **Explore Various Networks:** Leverage a combination of in-person groups, online communities, mentors, and professional help for comprehensive support.
- **Engage Actively:** Participate regularly, share openly, and contribute to maximize the benefits of your support net-

works.

- **Utilize Technology:** Embrace digital tools and platforms to enhance connectivity and access to resources.
- **Overcome Challenges:** Address barriers like time constraints and stigma with proactive strategies and self-compassion.
- **Expand Support Horizons:** Incorporate additional support systems beyond ADHD to foster a balanced and enriched life.

By thoughtfully building and nurturing your support network, you empower yourself to navigate the complexities of ADHD with resilience, confidence, and community.

12

Thriving with ADHD: Embracing Strengths and Future Planning

Introduction: Redefining ADHD Beyond Challenges

Attention Deficit Hyperactivity Disorder (ADHD) has long been perceived predominantly through the lens of its challenges and symptoms. However, as understanding deepens, so does the recognition of the unique strengths and potentials that often accompany ADHD. For women navigating life with ADHD, embracing these strengths can transform perceived limitations into avenues for success and fulfillment. This chapter explores how women can harness their inherent talents, set meaningful goals, and plan strategically for a prosperous future. Through inspiring success stories and actionable strategies, we aim to shift the narrative from merely managing ADHD to thriving with it.

Embracing ADHD-Associated Strengths

ADHD is frequently associated with difficulties in attention regulation, impulsivity, and hyperactivity. However, alongside these challenges lie a host of strengths that, when recognized and nurtured, can be significant assets in various aspects of life.

Creativity and Innovation

One of the most celebrated strengths among individuals with ADHD is their creativity. The ability to think outside the box, connect seemingly unrelated ideas, and approach problems from unconventional angles can lead to groundbreaking innovations and artistic achievements.

Case Study: Emma's Artistic Journey

Emma, a graphic designer diagnosed with ADHD in her late twenties, initially struggled in structured corporate environments. Traditional workflows and rigid deadlines felt restrictive, stifling her creative expression. However, upon embracing her ADHD-driven creativity, Emma transitioned to freelancing. This shift allowed her to design on her terms, leading to a burgeoning portfolio that attracted high-profile clients. Emma's story illustrates how leveraging creative strengths can lead to both professional success and personal satisfaction.

Hyperfocus: A Double-Edged Sword Turned Asset

Hyperfocus, the ability to intensely concentrate on a task, is often seen as a challenge when it hinders shifting attention to other responsibilities. However, when directed purposefully, hyperfocus can lead to exceptional productivity and mastery in specific areas.

Personal Anecdote: Sarah's Coding Marathon

Sarah, a software developer with ADHD, discovered her hyperfocus during a critical project deadline. Instead of viewing it as an uncontrollable distraction, she learned to channel this intense concentration into coding marathons. By structuring her work sessions around her natural periods of hyperfocus, Sarah not only met her project goals but also significantly contributed to innovative features within her company's software. This deliberate harnessing of hyperfocus transformed a potential obstacle into a career-defining strength.

Resilience and Adaptability

Women with ADHD often develop remarkable resilience and adaptability as they navigate a world that doesn't always accommodate their unique ways of thinking and processing. These traits foster perseverance, problem-solving abilities, and the capacity to thrive in dynamic environments.

Case Study: Laura's Entrepreneurial Spirit

Laura, an entrepreneur diagnosed with ADHD in her thirties, embarked on launching a tech startup after multiple unsuccessful ventures. Her ADHD-fueled adaptability allowed her to pivot business strategies swiftly in response to market feedback. Despite the unpredictability and challenges, Laura's resilience kept her motivated and engaged. Her startup eventually succeeded, becoming a recognized player in the tech industry. Laura's journey underscores how resilience and adaptability, honed through living with ADHD, are invaluable assets in the entrepreneurial landscape.

Setting Meaningful Goals: Aligning with Strengths and Passions

Setting goals is a fundamental aspect of personal and professional growth. For women with ADHD, the process of goal-setting requires a nuanced approach that aligns with their strengths, interests, and intrinsic motivations.

Identifying Passion-Driven Goals

Passion fuels perseverance. Women with ADHD often thrive when pursuing goals that resonate deeply with their interests and passions. Identifying what genuinely excites and motivates them can lead to more sustained effort and greater satisfaction.

Personal Anecdote: Mia's Passion for Environmental Advocacy

Mia, a marketing manager with ADHD, found herself constantly restless in her role, seeking greater purpose. She realized her passion lay in environmental advocacy. By setting a goal to integrate sustainable practices into her company's marketing strategies, Mia not only revitalized her professional life but also contributed meaningfully to a cause she cared about. Her alignment of goals with personal passion exemplifies how meaningful objectives can drive both career satisfaction and personal fulfillment.

SMART Goal Framework with ADHD Considerations

The SMART framework—Specific, Measurable, Achievable, Relevant, Time-bound—provides a structured approach to goal-setting. For women with ADHD, incorporating flexibility and adaptability into this framework can enhance its effectiveness.

- **Specific:** Clearly define what you want to achieve.
- **Measurable:** Establish criteria to track progress.
- **Achievable:** Ensure the goal is realistic given your resources and constraints.
- **Relevant:** Align the goal with your broader aspirations and strengths.
- **Time-bound:** Set a clear timeline to maintain focus and motivation.

Case Study: Nina's Career Advancement Plan

Nina, a project manager with ADHD, aimed to secure a leadership position within her company. Applying the SMART framework, she set a specific goal to complete a leadership training program within six months (Specific, Measurable, Time-bound). She ensured the goal was achievable by seeking employer support and dedicating regular time slots for training (Achievable). The goal was relevant as it aligned with her aspiration to lead teams effectively (Relevant). By monitoring her progress monthly, Nina maintained focus and ultimately earned a promotion, demonstrating the practical application of SMART goals enhanced for ADHD considerations.

Personal Growth and Self-Actualization

Thriving with ADHD involves continual personal growth and the pursuit of self-actualization. Embracing one's ADHD traits as integral parts of identity can foster a sense of empowerment and purpose.

Building Self-Awareness

Understanding personal strengths, weaknesses, triggers, and patterns is crucial for growth. Self-awareness enables women with ADHD to make informed decisions, set appropriate boundaries, and seek environments that nurture their potential.

Personal Anecdote: Jasmine's Journey to Self-Discovery

Jasmine, a freelance writer with ADHD, embarked on a journey of self-discovery after years of feeling out of place in traditional work settings. Through journaling and mindfulness practices, she gained deeper insights into her creative processes and energy cycles. This self-awareness allowed Jasmine to optimize her work schedule, prioritize tasks that aligned with her strengths, and develop strategies to mitigate distractions. Her enhanced self-knowledge not only improved her productivity but also bolstered her confidence and sense of purpose.

Cultivating a Growth Mindset

A growth mindset—the belief that abilities and intelligence can be developed—can significantly impact how women with ADHD approach challenges and opportunities. Embracing a growth mindset encourages resilience, continuous learning, and adaptability.

Case Study: Olivia's Pursuit of Continuous Learning

Olivia, an educator with ADHD, faced setbacks when her initial teaching methods did not resonate with her students. Instead of viewing these setbacks as failures, Olivia adopted a growth mindset, seeing them as opportunities to refine her techniques. She pursued professional development courses, sought mentorship, and experimented with innovative teaching strategies. Olivia's commitment to growth and learning transformed her teaching practice, leading to improved student outcomes and professional recognition.

Strategic Future Planning: Charting a Path Forward

Future planning involves envisioning where you want to be and outlining the steps to get there. For women with ADHD, strategic planning entails balancing ambition with flexibility, setting realistic milestones, and anticipating potential obstacles.

Vision Boarding and Visualization Techniques

Creating a visual representation of goals can help in clarifying aspirations and maintaining focus. Vision boards and visualization techniques are powerful tools for materializing intentions and reinforcing commitment.

Personal Anecdote: Lily's Vision Board Success

Lily, an aspiring architect with ADHD, utilized vision boarding to map out her career aspirations. By visually representing her goals—such as enrolling in a specialized architecture program, securing internships, and eventually designing sustainable buildings—Lily maintained a clear focus on her objectives. The tangible representation of her dreams provided daily motivation and a sense of direction, ultimately guiding her through the necessary steps to achieve her professional ambitions.

Time Management and Organization Strategies

Effective time management and organizational skills are pivotal for achieving long-term goals. Women with ADHD can employ specialized strategies to enhance their planning and execution processes.

Case Study: Hannah's Structured Scheduling

Hannah, a novelist with ADHD, struggled with managing her writing schedule amidst numerous distractions. She adopted a structured scheduling approach, allocating specific time blocks for writing, research, and revision. Utilizing digital calendars with reminders and breaking down projects into manageable tasks, Hannah significantly improved her productivity. This structured approach not only facilitated the completion of her novel but also instilled a sense of accomplishment and progress.

Leveraging Technology and Tools

Modern technology offers a plethora of tools designed to aid in goal-setting, time management, and organization. Leveraging these resources can enhance efficiency and support sustained progress.

Personal Anecdote: Zoe's Tech-Enhanced Productivity

Zoe, a digital marketer with ADHD, integrated various technological tools into her daily routine to manage her tasks and deadlines. Utilizing project management apps like Trello, digital note-taking tools like Evernote, and time-tracking software like Toggl, Zoe streamlined her workflow and minimized distractions. These tools provided her with visual task boards, seamless access to notes, and real-time tracking of her productivity, enabling her to stay organized and focused on her goals.

Building a Supportive Environment

Thriving with ADHD is not solely an individual endeavor; it often requires a supportive environment that fosters growth and accommodates unique needs. Building such an environment involves cultivating supportive relationships, seeking professional guidance, and creating conducive physical and emotional spaces.

Fostering Supportive Relationships

Having a network of understanding and supportive individuals can significantly impact one's ability to thrive with ADHD. Whether it's family, friends, mentors, or professional networks, these relationships provide encouragement, accountability, and practical assistance.

Case Study: Maya's Mentorship Experience

Maya, a graphic designer with ADHD, sought mentorship to navigate her career challenges. Partnering with a seasoned professional who understood her ADHD traits, Maya received tailored advice, feedback, and encouragement. The mentor helped her identify her strengths, set achievable goals, and develop strategies to overcome obstacles. This mentorship not only accelerated Maya's career growth but also enhanced her self-confidence and resilience.

Seeking Professional Guidance

Engaging with healthcare professionals, coaches, and therapists can provide invaluable support for managing ADHD and achieving personal growth. These professionals offer specialized strategies, coping mechanisms, and personalized plans to aid in thriving with ADHD.

Personal Anecdote: Rachel's Therapeutic Journey

Rachel, a teacher with ADHD, sought the assistance of a cognitive-behavioral therapist to address her challenges with time management and organization. Through therapy, Rachel developed practical strategies such as prioritizing tasks, setting realistic deadlines, and implementing organizational systems. The professional guidance she received empowered Rachel to improve her classroom management, reduce stress, and enhance her overall well-being, illustrating the profound impact of professional support.

Creating Conducive Physical and Emotional Spaces

Designing environments that minimize distractions and promote focus can significantly enhance productivity and well-being. Additionally, cultivating emotional spaces that nurture mental health is essential for thriving with ADHD.

Case Study: Anna's Optimized Home Office

Anna, a freelance writer with ADHD, transformed her home office into a distraction-free zone by incorporating organizational tools, ergonomic furniture, and soothing colors. She also established a daily routine that included regular breaks and relaxation techniques to maintain emotional balance. This optimized environment not only boosted her productivity but also fostered a sense of calm and creativity, enabling Anna to excel in her writing endeavors.

Future Planning: Long-Term Strategies for Success

Looking ahead requires proactive planning and the ability to adapt to changing circumstances. For women with ADHD, developing long-term strategies ensures sustained growth and the ability to navigate future challenges effectively.

Continuous Learning and Skill Development

Commitment to lifelong learning and continual skill development is crucial for staying relevant and competitive in an ever-evolving landscape. Women with ADHD can leverage their natural curiosity and adaptability to embrace new learning opportunities.

Personal Anecdote: Karen's Pursuit of Advanced Education

Karen, an operations manager with ADHD, recognized the importance of advanced skills in her field. She pursued a part-time Master's degree in Business Administration, utilizing strategies such as structured study schedules, interactive learning methods, and frequent breaks to manage her attention. Karen's dedication to continuous learning not only advanced her career but also kept her intellectually engaged and motivated.

Financial Planning and Stability

Financial stability is a cornerstone of long-term success and security. Women with ADHD can benefit from structured financial planning, including budgeting, saving, and investing, to ensure a stable future.

Case Study: Laura's Financial Management System

Laura, a single mother with ADHD, struggled with managing her finances due to impulsive spending and inconsistent budgeting. She adopted a comprehensive financial management system, utilizing budgeting apps, setting up automatic savings, and consulting with a financial advisor. By implementing these structured approaches, Laura achieved greater financial stability, reduced stress, and secured a futures fund for her children's education. Her story highlights the importance of strategic financial planning for long-term security.

Embracing Flexibility and Adaptability

The ability to adapt to unforeseen changes and remain flexible in the face of challenges is vital for sustained success. Women with ADHD can cultivate this trait by embracing change as an opportunity rather than a setback.

Personal Anecdote: Nina's Adaptive Career Path

Nina, a marketing specialist with ADHD, faced unexpected industry shifts that rendered her previous expertise less relevant. Instead of feeling defeated, Nina embraced the changes, seeking out new trends and acquiring skills in digital marketing analytics. Her adaptability enabled her to pivot her career successfully, securing a role in a cutting-edge marketing firm. Nina's experience underscores the value of flexibility and the willingness to embrace new opportunities.

Conclusion: Embracing a Thriving Future

Thriving with ADHD involves a transformative journey of self-discovery, strategic planning, and the celebration of unique strengths. For women with ADHD, recognizing and harnessing their innate talents—such as creativity, hyperfocus, resilience, and adaptability—can unlock pathways to personal and professional fulfillment. By setting meaningful goals, fostering supportive environments, and employing long-term strategies, women with ADHD can transcend societal stereotypes and redefine success on their own terms.

This chapter serves as a testament to the potential that lies within each woman with ADHD. Embracing these strengths not only enhances individual lives but also contributes to diverse and innovative communities. As society continues to evolve in its understanding of ADHD, the narrative shifts from one of limitation to one of empowerment and possibility. By embracing their ADHD-associated strengths and strategically planning for the future, women with ADHD can truly thrive, leaving indelible marks in their chosen fields and inspiring others along the way.

Additional Resources

To further support your journey in thriving with ADHD, consider exploring the following resources:

- **Books:**
- *Driven to Distraction* by Edward M. Hallowell and John J. Ratey
- *You Mean I'm Not Lazy, Stupid or Crazy?!* by Kate Kelly and Peggy Ramundo
- **Websites:**
- CHADD (Children and Adults with Attention-Deficit/Hyper activity Disorder): www.chadd.org
- ADDitude Magazine: www.additudemag.com

- **Apps:**
- Trello: Project management tool to organize tasks and collaborate.
- Evernote: Note-taking app to capture and organize ideas.
- Toggl: Time-tracking software to monitor productivity.
- **Support Groups:**
- Women with ADHD Facebook Groups: Connect with a community of women sharing similar experiences.
- Local CHADD Chapters: Engage with local support groups and events.

By leveraging these resources, you can continue to build a supportive network, gain new insights, and access tools that facilitate your journey towards thriving with ADHD.

In embracing their strengths and strategically planning for the future, women with ADHD are not only overcoming challenges but are also setting new standards for what it means to live a fulfilling and successful life. The journey is unique for each individual, but the shared experiences and collective wisdom empower women to navigate their paths with confidence, resilience, and an unwavering commitment to their personal growth and aspirations.

Here are some book title options for **"The Definitive Guide to ADHD for Women"**:

1. **"ADHD and Me: A Woman's Guide to Understanding and Thriving"**
2. **"Empowered with ADHD: A Woman's Journey Through Diagnosis and Beyond"**

3. **"Unlocking Potential: The Comprehensive Guide to ADHD in Women"**
4. **"ADHD Uncovered: Navigating Life and Relationships as a Woman"**
5. **"She Focuses Too: A Woman's Path to Managing ADHD with Confidence"**
6. **"Beyond the Stereotypes: Empowering Women with ADHD"**
7. **"The ADHD Women's Handbook: Strategies for Life and Love"**
8. **"ADHD through Her Lens: A Guide for Women Seeking Answers"**
9. **"Resilient Minds: Thriving with ADHD as a Woman"**
10. **"Living Loudly: A Woman's Definitive Guide to Empowering Your ADHD Experience"**

Each title aims to resonate with the experiences of women dealing with ADHD while conveying empowerment and support.